THE FOURTH QUARTER

The Hail Mary for Seniors

Dede Weldon Casad, Ph.D.

Copyright © 2013 Dede Weldon Casad, Ph.D.

All rights reserved.

Get information about Dede Casad's other books at

www.DedeCasad.com

Contents

Acknowledgements v

Preface vii

THE MISSION: Making the Most of the Fourth Quarter 1

THE LINEUP: Introducing the First String—My Support Group ... 3

THE SCORE BOARD: Evaluating Your Value to the Game of Life 23

CALL THE PLAY: Joining the Game and Making it Your Passion 37

FATE or DESTINY: Playing the Whole Field 49

CALL TIME: Recognizing the Sense of Urgency 55

THE WIDE RECEIVER: Opening Up to the Opportunities 67

THE HAIL MARY: Eyeing the Ticking Time Clock 91

THE FINAL SCORE: Crossing the Goal Line with Personal Satisfaction 103

About the Author 121

Acknowledgements

This book is dedicated to the coffee group at the mall. Each person has a special place in my friendship folder. For over 20 years, the group has entertained me, corrected me, endured my right brain flare-ups, tolerated the many off-the-wall questions, and yet supported me anyway.

You have been great!

Preface

I am on a mission. And I am recruiting missionaries. I don't want to do this by myself. I want to gather a crowd and start out together in the hope that the trail behind us will be as endless as time itself. If you are 65, and wondering about how best to spend your final years, or if you are in your seventies and retirement isn't as glamorous as you had hoped, or if you are in your eighties and thinking about leaving a legacy, then join me. Join my mission. Together we can kiss the blarney stone and change the cultural imbalance in the world.

Ours is a high-level, blue-ribbon, individually gratifying, industrial-sized mission; a mission designed specifically and deliberately for people past the prime of life who are refusing to take aging lying down—no pun intended. Senior citizens are survivors, a select group, a chosen people, and being a survivor means you have been hand-picked, unequivocally selected and earmarked for special assignments. As blessed people who are living ten or twenty years longer than the actuarial age charts suggest, we find ourselves in the enviable position of being eye-witness to history, as custodians of valuable stories, lessons, and information, and as guardians of a collective wisdom gathered over three-fourths of a century. Our mission is to determine our personal goals first, then help others realize the obligation we all have to the world to give back a portion of what we have received in life, in response to the scriptural passage, "For to whom much is given, much is required." In addition, our mission is to motivate seniors not to give up living, but to make their latter days purposefully joyful with a meaning that matters, and then to inspire them to finish with a MAD (Making a Difference) dash to the goal line, proudly standing tall.

I call this mission…The Fourth Quarter.

THE MISSION:
Making the Most of the Fourth Quarter

Most Americans have bought into the concept that when we retire, we deserve a life of leisure. Where did we get that idea? Never in the history of humankind has a culture embraced such a non-productive, valueless philosophy as wholeheartedly as have Americans. The rapid development of retirement communities, rest homes, and assisted living facilities in the last thirty years bears testimony to the fact that Americans have adopted this viewpoint with their mind, money, and minimum objection. Just read the retirement village's advertisements in the newspapers. *The Life You've Dreamed About; Great Golf Courses for Everyone—Come Enjoy our Leisurely Way of Life.* If we didn't believe we deserved leisure in retirement before, the advertising moguls are continually trying to convince us that we do.

Yes, we have been convinced it is time to take down our shingles, put up a do-not-disturb sign, and tell everyone glibly, "I get up every morning with nothing to do and go to bed with it half done." That's the American way. I am retired. I have worked my butt off for decades. Now I am going to buy me a rocking chair and rock my way into heaven.

If this is your mantra, I want you on my team, pronto. I want the person who honestly believes that retirement means a long holiday. I want the person who says "give me a fishing pole and watch me." I want the person who has put books back on the shelf, pots and pans deep under the sink, and sits and waits for the mailman to bring the bills. I also want that person who has tried this type of retirement and is beginning to realize that idle, useless retirement may not be all it is cracked up to be. It is lonely. It is boring, and it is often disappointing.

I want the people who have left the field of play; those who are sitting on the sideline of life, just waiting for the great coach in the sky to give them the nod that the game is over. If you are one of these people:

Come along. I need you.

Let's huddle.

THE FOURTH QUARTER

THE LINEUP:
Introducing the First String—My Support Group

Beautiful young people are accidents of nature, but beautiful old people are works of art. —Eleanor Roosevelt

Pregame Review

As a writer I am often asked where I get my ideas for a book. Generally, I just tell them, "everywhere." However, the idea for this book came from a source so close to home that I almost overlooked it. I had thought that the source was too familiar for me to consider their input fresh and relevant. But, I was dead wrong. They were exactly what I needed. They have all the components needed for a book about retirement, lifestyle, continuity, passion, calling, and destiny. They are my walking, talking, coffee group that meets every morning except Sunday and has done so continuously for more than 15 years.

Through the years, the group has added and subtracted members as death and life situations intervened. Today, from our original 18 members, we are now down to 11.

The group comprises four men and seven women who are all heavily into their fourth quarter, representing a microcosm of the huge pool of senior citizens living in America today. What has kept us together these many years is an invisible camaraderie cord that none of us can fully identify or explain. We are dissimilar as to our past, our personalities, our life's work, and our world views. One might never expect any of us to have a social relationship with the other. Also, one might suspect that after 15 years, we might drift apart, seek friendships elsewhere, or stop attending the meet-up all together. But no, we get up every morning with the deliberate intention of going to the mall for coffee (walking has long since become a maybe-tomorrow activity for most of us). Unless Roxie has to man the food distribution center, or Lucy has to attend a board meeting, or Ralph is off holding a seminar in Utah, or Chuck has to attend one of his military meetings, or Janet has to meet with her broker, or Reed and Jane have to go to their lake house, or Frances and Marion have to flit to Las Vegas to gamble, or Bob has to grade graduate papers, most of us show up.

We are not a shabby lot. Indeed, professionally, we represent a comfortable mix of occupational expertise, from a housewife and an artist, to a geologist, medical scientist, financial planner, tax authority, teacher, writer, military officer, and a high level public economist.

However, diverse as we are, we have a common thread that weaves us together—we are all avid readers. To find another commonality might be like searching for the proverbial needle in a haystack.

Most of us are computer savvy. In the last fifteen years we have moved from landlines to cell phones, iPhones, iPods, and Androids; from handwritten letters to fax and emails, and from shopping in stores to online shopping. We are not stymied by new technology. We will not allow it to get ahead of us, lest we fall too far behind to ever catch up. We refuse to stay in the dark about what is new in computer software, phone service apps, or innovative offers from AT&T, Verizon, Sprint, or Apple. Even though most of us do not truly understand the inner workings of these modern marvels, we spend a good amount of time helping each other resolve computer glitches, reconfiguring cell phones, adding new apps, and sharing what news there might be concerning the latest technical toys. When one of our machines falters, suggestions for solutions make the rounds. Usually, it's Janet or Bob who ends up giving the right answer. Trading information about apps causes us to whip out our cell phones and begin downloading. Everyone wants Dragon and the new voice-activated Google, and of course, we want to get in on the ground floor of 'Word with Friends.'

On any given day, as soon as we have resolved the immediate technical exchanges, the conversation invariably turns to sports or politics. If there has been a football game the night before, the discussion of the game takes over for the next 30 or 40 minutes, then we're off onto politics. Local news has to be fairly dramatic to get coverage at the coffee table because we replay CNN and FOX breaking news almost verbatim the next morning.

When we are all in attendance, all eleven are seated around one table with some members straddling the corner legs. This more than doubles the normal occupancy of the table that is set for four. Ralph sets the stage. He is usually the first to arrive and he determines, among the twenty or so available tables in the middle of the mall adjoining *la Madeleine's,* where we sit. Being square in the middle of the mall with aisles on both sides of us is a perfect place for people watching and commenting. We observe people walking by and remark about outlandish hairdos, disgraceful t-shirts, short skirts, adorable babies, and rude mothers who push strollers butt-up against our table. We have been mall regulars so long that the mall manager often stops by to give us an update on new stores opening and old ones closing. We watch as the florist changes floral decorations from lilies in April to poinsettias in December. We watch as the local car dealers roll their most luxurious cars into the mall for show and tell. We know exactly when the *Race for the Cure* is due, the Playhouse contest will be held and the schedule of the bi-yearly art show. Of course, we look forward to seeing the toy train exhibit and Santa Claus at Christmas.

All of this and more is the morning experience of the coffee group. When we have exhausted the gauntlet of news and gossip we reluctantly say goodbye for the day.

I have several reasons for introducing the group. First, we are all senior citizens, retired and still actively involved. Second, we consider ourselves still vital, energetic, mentally astute, well-read, highly intelligent, and fun. We also have the basic characteristics of people prepared to live to one hundred years of age. Our attitudes are positive, our lifestyles tempered and settled, and we have the financial means to see us to the end. We also have a combination of intellectual vision and creative know-how to illustrate that anyone can make a difference in this world.

More to the point, each of us, in one form or another, is still contributing. We have not given up the game. We are scoring points and, in fact, are decidedly engaged and involved in the affairs of the community.

Describing these friends is difficult. There is no hierarchy, no rank or rating we could use, no alphabetical system or age distinction to designate or classify an adequate lineup. Each one deserves his or her special place and anyone could easily be first. But here we go.

Reed and Jane Pierce represent the best of us all. They are genuine fun-loving people. Jane, with her undiluted laughter, is noncritical and totally without guile. The worker-helper type, Jane is the kind of friend everyone wants as she brings joy along with her. Reed, on the other hand, even with a smile on his face and a twinkle in his eyes, is short on patience when it comes to electronics or difficult to understand voices on the telephone. His tolerance level is somewhere between not much and nothing at all when it comes to car dealerships, outboard motor repairs, and tree removal or computer foul-ups. Owner of all major technical equipment, Reed fights the breakdown battle with vengeance. He worked for Exxon Mobil for over 40 years as the Western Regional Manager of property tax, a complicated enterprise at best. His real claim on our hearts, however, is also one that endears him to thousands of Americans; Reed is a national hero. He was shot down over Germany in WWII and lived to tell the most fascinating stories of survival as a prisoner of war. When Reed and Jane joined our coffee group they had a home in Dallas, two lake houses, and her mother's home under their care and supervision. The incredible job of keeping four houses running smoothly along with attending ailing extended family members has taken most of their retirement time. However, they have traveled globally and amassed friends from all over the world.

Reed and Jane are three days a week coffee table regulars, leaving days at home for a thousand chores that, at ages 92 and 78 respectively, they are still capable of doing. When Reed and Jane are at coffee shop, the enjoyment rises appreciably.

Roxie McIntyre is a retired physical therapist, and—oh boy, is she called on to diagnose any new ache or pain! She knows every muscle, tendon, and joint and their respective potential disorders. Her advice and counsel on anything related to the physical ache has saved most of us from orthopedic appointments and chiropractor's adjustments. She now lives alone in a house that sits on a piece of property that would make her wealthy, but wealth is not her goal. Roxie's home is as much a part of her as the furniture in it. In fact, she built most of it herself! She and her friend Maggie took woodworking classes in an old Dallas school and learned how to make furniture. Her home has one-of-a-kind bedstead, dresser, and end tables; all especially carved, sanded, stained and beautifully finished to her specifications.

The coffee group often gravitates around Roxie because she is a natural born wit. Her sense of humor cuts through our conversations, clearing up heated conversations at just the right moment, and giving us all a welcomed laugh of comic relief. The other day, for instance, when thunder clouds were all around, one of us remarked that he had gotten over an inch of rain, while another said she hadn't gotten a drop. Roxie piped up innocently, "Well, I got two inches of thunder." None of us could top that.

Lucy is our teacher. She taught the third grade for over 30 years, first in Nebraska and then in Dallas. Teacher-like, she uses the pedagogy technique when making a statement by punctuating her point with an index finger. This is her way of holding the group's attention for the moment. An ardent football fan, Lucy is knowledgeable about players and coaches and has a plus or minus opinion about each of them as she banters back and forth with Ralph and Chuck about sports. The three of them make quite a news reel reenacting plays as Monday morning quarterbacks. Being from Pierce, Nebraska, Lucy believes there is only one good football team: the one from the University of Nebraska.

Well-read and well-versed in the latest political controversy, Lucy quotes the newspaper and the latest attention-getting comments from her favorite television channel. Very little goes by Lucy, unnoticed or undocumented. She speaks with authority and resolve and has yet to risk looking at Snopes, to verify if fiction is disguised as fact on some of the many emails that flood our inboxes daily.

Ralph is our Ph.D. of record. Now retired as Chief Geologist of Exxon Mobil, Ralph is still in high demand for lectures, consulting, and holding field trips for oil companies around the world. Likewise, he is generally up on sports, but there is no one in the group that can match his knowledge about gourmet restaurants. He also follows with great interest the noted chefs of our city. He and Janet both have taken several gourmet cooking courses and have become our consultants on the best wines to buy. Thanks to their gracious hospitality, their home is the ideal party house for any holiday.

Ralph is slow to comment. And as a man of few words, he relies on others to initiate the discussion, and then replies when directly asked. He sits at the head of the table and acts as host for the occasion. His is also the best seat for people watching and reporting.

Janet is our investment expert and financial planner. She listens and watches the Bloomberg report every morning, and checks the market and manages her own portfolio. As she says, "Ralph brought home the paycheck, but I make the money." Janet is perhaps the most well-rounded person of the group. She cooks, she gardens, she plays intellectual games, and she volunteers at the children's hospital as the 'popcorn lady,' serving patients and their families. If she has flaws, they are deeply hidden from us because we sincerely admire her marvelous attitude. She is also the least healthy one of the bunch. She suffers from crippling arthritis and is rarely without pain. She never complains. She will say where she hurts, but she doesn't dwell on her aches and pains; in fact, she strives at working through it with all she's got. Her love is her grandson, Conner, whom we have all adopted as our own, even though most of us have grandsons as well.

Frances and Marion have been close friends since their college years and have shared their lives as friends. Frances is a histotechnologist and Marion is an artist. Few people know what a histotechnologist is, but when you find out that Frances, with a Ph.D. in chemistry, has written the seminal text book on the subject, you realize what an unusual and remarkable person she is. Frances's job of analyzing the tissue slides for surgeons to determine how they are to proceed is always critical to the well-being of the patient.

Marion, on the other hand, has made her living as an artist, most notably as a watercolor artist. Her paintings hang on many walls in Dallas homes as treasured works of art. How different these two women are, yet how compatible. They say art and science can never mesh, but theirs is a perfect example of blending and cooperation between right and left brain people.

Frances could double for a queen in the Elizabethan era. She stands regally and proud. Her hair is cropped close to her head and carefully groomed. Not a hair is ever out of place. When she first joined the group, she had little to say, yet over time she has become one of the most articulate of all the members.

As I mentioned, Marion has made a name for herself in the Dallas art community. Like most artist I know, though I hate to generalize, she has a soft touch, a calm voice and an easy manner that expresses itself with a smile that will melt your heart. The people she meets never stay a stranger for long; she is often the first one to talk to others sitting at nearby tables. If you want a friend, Marion more than qualifies.

Bob is our newest member and perhaps the most interdisciplinary intellectual of the bunch. He is also the only one not officially retired. Coming from a financial background, he is bombarded with questions from the group about the economic conditions of our country. He is quick to respond, and explains the most complicated economic situations with clarity and authority. As a single man with three grown children, he has perfected the art of living alone. He is a gourmet cook with an entire closet devoted to cooking utensils. Nothing is beyond his epicurean interest. The other day, he was telling us how he made marmalade. No one else around that table had ever considered making marmalade, for heaven's sake, yet Bob spent two days creating a divine batch that he graciously shared with the group. With extensive experience in both the private and public sector of the economic world, Bob spends months consulting with third world countries concerning monetary policies and keeps us up-to-date on multicultural and international developments.

That leaves Chuck and me.

In a later chapter I will tell you about us, but to know Chuck is to know one great guy. Chuck was a B-24 pilot during World War II, having flown 36 missions over Germany. After the war, he chose to remain in the Air Force as a career officer. His military life placed him in strategic places worldwide; he is the quintessential world citizen. His patriotism and love of America has stayed with him through the years as he continues to champion all military efforts. He maintains contact not only with his former crewmen, but with men across America as well who were part of the 2nd Air Division during the war.

So, ignoring for the moment the obvious, that our group sits on our butts for a good hour each morning, we nonetheless represent a legitimate cross-section of Fourth Quarter people attempting to make the most of the days we have left.

There is not a lazy person among us. Some have more natural energy than others and that level of energy defines the degree to which we are physically active. Since all of us are professionals, there is an intellectual give and take, tension and release, input and output springing back and forth every morning. There is competition and compromise. There is criticism and praise. There is occasional good-will and ill-will, but none of this seems to sabotage our care or appreciation for one another. What keeps us together is the miracle that becomes clearer as we mush along.

When I asked each person in my group why they keep coming to coffee, or why they chose to stay with the group, I was forced on the spot to answer my own question. I told them that I return, not so much out of habit, although there is an element of that, but in order to continue to stimulate my interpersonal skills and love for debate. The group provides a forum, a stage if you will, for performing and renewing the ability to communicate, to clarify my opinions as well as discover when I am wrong, which is important to me. Meeting with these people every day forces me to think outside myself, my own self-interests, and my own pet projects.

After I confessed why I continue to come to coffee, the group loosened up and began to think about their own motives. Janet said she comes because we have created a strong support group—which, of course, is true. We have lost three members by death and each of us was a part of their illnesses and final loss. We took them to the hospitals, drove them to therapy, and then finally joined them at their funerals.

When I asked Lucy why she comes, I had to supply a reason why I asked before she would answer. Evidently, Lucy needed a starting point and wanted to be sure she was lined up in agreement with the group before committing herself.

Janet mentioned we might be too homogeneous and noted that we simply exchange information we read or heard on television the night before. When we talk about politics, she pointed out that some of us merely regurgitate what O'Reilly, Hannity, Greta, Blitzer, or Anderson Cooper had said the night before. Janet hates that!

Frances was quick with a single, concise answer to my question—"sociability." Crisp and honest and to the point. Then Marion added a very provocative addendum— "This group is my family. I do not have children and you are my family."
I was stunned. It would never have occurred to me that the group could be considered 'family.' This opened my eyes to how differently each of us perceives the group. Those of us with children could not have come close to a remark such as Marion's, but she sized it up succinctly. You have to love it.

As we proceed, the group will be part of the discussions that follow. Some in the coffee group seem to like the fact that I am writing a book about Fourth Quarter people, and their role in it. Others, admittedly, are more reserved. However, I guarantee their input will prove fun, insightful, and definitely helpful.

Coaches

Before we start talking about our Fourth Quarter mission, some coaching is required. If nothing else, we must look at aging in a new way and evaluate the aging culture and how we are affected by it. Some of us may also need an attitude adjustment about how we feel about growing older.

There are coaches for every known human situation. There are defensive coaches, offensive coaches, business coaches, life coaches, management coaches, and leadership coaches, just to name a few. Each one has his particular expertise for a particular function of human endeavor. Our need is for an aging coach to prepare us and then place us properly on the field of play.

An aging coach tells us there are more than forty million people over the age of 65 in America today. That's a lot of company we have. Even more startling is the fact that there are more than 71,000 Americans over the age of 100. Experts say this number will reach 241,000 by 2020, because of the baby boomers. Starting next year, these boomers arrive in staggering numbers. Let's allow others to deal with the Social Security issue while we will deal with the practical questions and subsequent changes these figures represent.

If the rumors are true that 60 is the new 40 and 70 is the new 50, those of us now in the Fourth Quarter must modify our thinking about how we spend the rest of our lives. To consider living thirty years after retirement forces us to reevaluate and then reconstruct our future. The old stereotypes about aging are no longer applicable. Pneumonia is no longer the death knell of 50 years ago. The word 'infirm' has dropped from the Fourth Quarter lexicon. Driver's licenses are still issued to many citizens over the age of 90. The idea that older people have lost their power is totally and unequivocally untrue.

Today, the age wave is a tsunami causing a complete reversal of old views about aging. Marketing experts are quickly changing the image of 'age' to 'lifestyle' and from touting youth to respecting the wise. Age is not a four-letter word. In fact, many pundits believe that this age wave of thoughtful, patriotic seniors, who are continuing to offer their opinions and exercise their right to vote, will be a major political factor in the coming presidential elections.

Individually and collectively, Fourth Quarter people are rendering more power now than ever before.

My mission is to waken seniors to that reality, motivate them to use their power wisely, and inspire them to spend the rest of their lives making a difference. No longer can we say, 'I'm just one person, what can I do?' The world is full of individuals making huge contributions every minute of every day.

Paul Harvey continued his radio broadcast and tells listeners the 'rest of the story' until he died at 88.

Millicent Fenwick, from New Jersey, ran for Congress and served for eight years after she was 70. She became affectionately known, by her fellow congressmen, as the 'the conscious of the Congress.'

Timing and the current culture is on our side. Half of all the people who have ever lived to age 65 are currently alive. That's you and me. Soon there will be more senior citizens than children. And coaches tell us that if we are now 65, we can expect to live to be 76. And while we can't use our backs as we once did, we can use our minds. While climbing stairs may be harder, we can easily tutor young people. While it may be more difficult to get out of the bathtub, we can certainly use the telephone to check on shut-ins.

Our bodies are unmistakably in worse shape than when we were 20, but these restrictions are more than compensated by our experience and know-how. Our joints no longer work as a well-oiled machine, our eyes no longer focus with 20/20 vision, our ears are clogged with more than beeswax and the dip stick tells us our energy levels are low. But here we are and we can continue to lag or we can rally the phagocytes, shake off the malaise, and with recharged batteries and a clear passion, make a difference.

So we ask ourselves, how old is old? When we do, we find advantages coming from everywhere. For instance, contrary to popular belief, statistics show that older people are victimized less;

have fewer car accidents than any other age groups; have fewer responsibilities for raising children; have lower rates of mental illness; and have more social freedom. On the giving side, older adults are more law abiding, vote and volunteer more regularly, and unlike the younger generation, have more wisdom to share.

Several years back, Green Thumb, Inc. launched the National Prime Time Awards Program to highlight valuable contributions older Americans make to their communities. Each year they search for the oldest worker in the country.

In 2011, Huda Bolger Becker won the award at the age of 102. She cofounded the Wright Institute in Los Angeles for mental health training. As a psychiatrist, she sees patients 16 to 20 hours a week, writes, gives lectures, and appears in professional videos.

Another winner was Mazarin Wingate at the age of 101. He started out as a custodian at the United States Post Office in Lexington, Kentucky and still works there four to six hours every day as well as driving himself to and from the office.

Ralph Eisenberg won the prize in 2000. He manages the California Zipper plant, still negotiates with vendors and clients, and services some of the company's longstanding accounts. He was 102 years of age.

Dr. William Sunderman won it in 1999. He was a world-renowned physician, pathologist, clinical scientist and chemist, and a lifelong violinist. He still gives concerts. He was 100 years old when he won.

Milt W. Garland won the prize in 1998. At age of 104 he went to the office every day, serving as Senior Consultant for Technical Services. He worked for the same firm that gave him his first job 81 years earlier.

Aging then must be redefined or even renamed. Maybe 'aging' is out and 'maturity' is in. Instead of considering the elderly useless and helpless, consider their power. Singly and collectively, we are commanding more attention, gaining more notoriety, making more money, and saving more than any generation before us. And for the first time, the marketing industry is beginning to realize this new and vital segment of our society and changing their marketing strategies to not only accommodate the over sixty-fives, but to appeal to their interest in a commercial way.

Equipment

I have a library in my home of more than 2,000 books. Some are as old as I am, but I can't part with them. One never knows when a given book holds just the right information or answer to a probing question; or waits patiently on the shelves to give me a boost of inspiration. Of course, many are reference books that I have used in planning or writing other books. Many of them are novels from favorite authors. I have an entire collection of books on writing, fewer than I once had because I often give one away in an attempt to encourage or help other writers. Some of my books have titles and authors I doubt you have ever heard of, while others have titles and authors that are as familiar to you as your street address. Books that surround my desk are religious and philosophical books which I have used in teaching Sunday school and relied upon for my own spiritual development.

I love my books and they love me back. I remember one of Leslie Conger's articles in *Writer's* magazine from years back. She wrote about her son preparing to go off to college. He was in her library and willy-nilly taking books off the shelves to take to school with him. Leslie said to him in a somewhat admonishing way, "Boy, take care of those books." She paused, and then said to herself privately, "Books take care of that boy."

I feel the same about my books. They are available to anyone who might want to borrow them, but to discard my books is simply not an option because they take care of me. They comfort me, they encourage me, they often confuse me and even rebuke me. They are my friends, my inspiration and most of all they are the source of my learning every day. My books and I are joined at the spine. Polling the coffee group about how they feel about books brought forth a discussion that should be noted here. Lucy, the elementary school teacher, loves her collection of children's books, especially those written by Tomie DePaola. She met Mr. DePaola at a book fair one day and he gave her a bookmark. Thinking how fine they were, Lucy asked him if she could have enough for her third grade students. DePaola asked if a hundred would be enough. Of course, she was thrilled and said "yes." Mr. DePaola stood there and counted out a hundred bookmarks for her. Lucy had them all laminated for permanent use and then passed out the bookmarks to her children. Children's books are a large part of her extensive library.

Jane told about the books that had been given to her and how emotionally attached she is to them. The inscriptions in the inside page make them hers and hers alone, and are part of her special treasury. These are never loaned out and will never be given away, so strong is her bond to them.

Chuck's books on World War II take up most of the shelving space in his library. Having flown out of the same air base in England with Jimmy Stewart, Chuck has a collection of Stewart biographies and his contributions to the war. And there has not been a book written about the B-24 airplane that Chuck does not have. One day he will send his books to Norwich, England, for permanent storage in the Second Air Division library and archives there.

Books matter to all of us.

This is not the Age of Aquarius.

This is the Age of Athena.

Principles of the Game

Markings by Dag Hammarskjold

For me, one of the most inspiring books is *Markings,* a book published long after the author died. Dag Hammarskjold was born in Sweden, the son of the Swedish prime minister serving during World War I. After studying law and economics, young Hammarskjold gained prominence as secretary and then chairman of the board of governors of the Bank of Sweden. Later he became undersecretary of the Swedish department of finance. In 1953 he was elected Secretary-General of the United Nations. Known around the world as a 'peacemaker,' Hammarskjold's writing avoids any mention of his personal career, but bears strongly on universal spiritual matters. Although he obtained great international success, his true devotion was to God and *Markings* captures his private thoughts and the deep revelations of his mind and spirit.

Markings was published posthumously after Hammarskjold died in a 1963 plane crash. But not until 1986 was the book translated into English and published in the United States by W. H. Auden. Since then, *Markings* has continued to be highly popular, with continuous interest by each new generation. And with good reason.

From the Sideline

Markings is a wisdom book. There is wisdom in almost every line. Along with the Bible, Thomas à Kempis' *The Imitation of Christ*, the Bhagavad-Gita, and some of C.S. Lewis' work, *Markings* is ageless. Wisdom books transcend time and territory, race and ideologies. If you are insightful, you can't miss the tremendous impact of Hammarskjold's thoughts. Some of his memorable lines include: "The present moment is significant, not as the bridge between past and future, but by reason of its contents, contents which can fill our emptiness and become ours, if we are capable of receiving them." Or this one, "At that moment came the certainty that existence is meaningful and that my life, therefore, in surrender, has a purpose." Or again, "Only when you descend into yourself and encounter the Other, do you then experience goodness as the ultimate reality—united and living—in Him and through you." Such beautiful and powerful insights speak across generations, across borders, and everyday thresholds. Wisdom filtered through to the soul for a searcher like you and me.

The other reason I am fond of Hammarskjold's work is because his writings helped lead my son, Vic, into the professional ministry in the United Methodist Church. Thus is the influence of words, and I can't help but wonder if any of the words I write or say could ever be that powerful. We will never know about any of the things we might say. We are totally unaware, most of the time, how or if God is using our words. The very thought of such power is awesome. But it does make us mindful of what we say and how we say it.

Words matter. We live by them. They motivate, they inspire. They teach, they scold and they create. They can also abuse or destroy. Like water or fire, words can be life-giving or life-taking. They can be harmful or helpful. But they are the only tools we use to express thoughts, write books, instruct and then, if need be, criticize. By words, we think, and from those words we respond and act.

One of my favorite words, which is only found in the Oxford Edition Dictionary, is *abecedarian*. The word rolls off the tongue like melted sugar as it describes a person teaching the ABCs in order to frame and form words. I have tried, in these few pages, to bring several types of word combinations, metaphorically through the game of football, to advance one single point—to encourage senior citizens to use their later years to fulfill their destiny. I have used books and their ideas, personal reflections and concrete examples to illustrate and encourage us to that end. The examples are sometimes famous people, but more often they are ordinary citizens doing extraordinary things that make a difference. I call these people, 'already in the game.'

To reinforce what wonderful things men and women can do after they retire, we remember George Burns, who played the leading role in the movies in *The Sunshine Boys* and *O God* in his late seventies and early eighties. His last film was *I Wish I Was 18 Again* when George was in his nineties. Oliver Wendell Holmes, who wrote *"Over the Teacups"* and Dick Van Dyke, who starred in the movie *A Night at the Museum,* or Jessica Tandy, who won an Oscar for her role in *Driving Miss Daisy* were into their eighties, and Marc Chagall, the first living artist to exhibit at the Louvre Museum in Paris. He was ninety at the time.

Granted these are famous people, but they made themselves memorable even in their later years. To paraphrase Gore Vidal, we will remember many famous people kindly until we forget, which we will in time, but we will remember these longer because they stayed in the game of life, playing all the way to the end.

As we progress through this book, we will learn about many people who are making a difference because they didn't say to themselves, "What can one person do?" Or, "I'm too old." They never considered their ages, but rather their opportunities and realized that their lives had a purpose and a destiny. That's you. That's also me.

Dr. Karl Pillemer, head of the Cornell Institute for Translational Research on Aging, has started what he calls *The Legacy Project: Lessons for Living from the Wisest Americans.* He believes in the wisdom of the elderly. One of his clients, Verna, who is 91 years old, wrote the following 'list for living' for her great-grandchildren. No greater legacy could she leave for the younger generation.

TO ALL MY WONDERFUL GREAT-GRANDCHILDREN—ALL OF THEM

1. So many things in the world have changed since the time of my grandparents and parents and the earlier times of my own life, and I know that there will be lots of changes in your lifetime, too.

2. I hope you will always take school seriously (I was a teacher) and become well-educated to be ready for whatever kind of work or service you will be doing; that you will respect your body—take good care of it and try to have good health.

3. I hope that the governments of the world will do a better job of getting along with each other so that you can experience peace among nations.

4. I hope you will be a positive thinker, not negative or cynical; look for the good in people and things, and fill your life with love, kindness, and thoughtfulness for others.

5. Most important is to know God as you go into the future. I would hope that you will know the peace and joy and courage that come from following a life of love and service—the peace that passes all understanding.

6. Your real success in life is the kind of person you become, not with how famous or wealthy you are, so my most sincere wish is for you to live the wholesome life that will lead you to make good choices along the way, to Reach that Star that you are striving to reach.

YOU CAN DO IT!

If Verna, at the age of 91, could write these valuable words for her great grandchildren, surely you can do no less. So suit up and get in the game.

THE SCORE BOARD:
Evaluating Your Value to the Game of Life

You know you're getting old when all the names in your black book have M.D. after them. — Arnold Palmer

What Counts

Looking at the scoreboard—we are shocked. The first three quarters have evaporated like raindrops and---oh my, we are behind. The clock is ticking. It's the fourth quarter. We are caught off-guard. Time is running out. We ask ourselves, can we still win this game of life? Is there still time for us to make a difference this close to the end of the game? And if so, how? What must we do to get across the goal line with the ball in our arms before the final whistle blows?

For those of us in the Fourth Quarter, these questions haunt us like the ghost of Christmas past. The end is drawing near. There is less time before us than behind us and weeks are flying by like days gobbling up precious moments. We feel an urgency to somehow, someway, score big. It is now or never.

Unfortunately, to move forward, we must take a brief glance backward, if only for a short visit. We don't want to get lost in nostalgia and lose more time, but it is important to quickly make an inventory. We'll call this practice time in preparation for the big game, because the past holds the play book for strategizing and executing the next play. We need the experiences of the past to understand the present before fulfilling our mission in the future.

So close the door and take out your pencil and start counting. Pull out the picture albums, the college yearbooks, old letters and address books, all those hand written data files you kept before the computer took over. Recall your first memory, you first love, your favorite pet. List the major decisions you made about jobs, marriage and major moves. Recall the losses and the hurts and again feel the pain. Spend a little time reviewing old pictures, saved scrapbook material, recipes, documents, lesson plans, flight schedules, diaries, journals, and trips.

List the people you have met along life's way. Recall the names of your teachers, your classmates, your team members, your fraternity or sorority buddies, your first boss, your first date. Remember your first pet, when he died, and how you felt. Remember the hardest thing you ever did and what you did wrong that you would never do again.

Remember the lessons your mother taught you, then the same for your father. Remember when you learned to swim or ride a bicycle and of course, the first thing you remember as a young child. Remember how you dressed when you were in grade school, high school and in college, even when you got your first long pants.

Remember what you thought you wanted to be when you grew up and what you finally did. Then remember your first girlfriend or boyfriend. Did that lead to your first love? What did you feel then? Did your parents approve of your choice? Remember the first heartache, the first accident, and the first loss of a family member or friend. Remember the first time you saw a dead person.

Check old Christmas cards for those who have now gone before you and ask what they meant to you at one time. Recall your reaction to Pearl Harbor or President Kennedy's assassination.

Include, of course, your marriage, where you went on your honeymoon. Remember why you choose him or her and the counseling session with your priest or minister before marriage. Recall the details of having your first child, the hospital experience, the grandparent's expressions, and those early days of sleepless nights.

Remember your first job, your boss's name and how he treated you, your college days and what you wish for then that did or did not pan out. Think of the places you have lived, the different houses and communities, the growing family responsibilities. Who did what around the house, who did the grocery buying and who attended the children's activities? Remember your favorite movie and movie stars. When your family got their first television set and what shows you watched as a family. Then lastly, remember what was important to you then, and what is important to you now.

Separately and collectively, your experiences count—the good ones, the bad ones, the funny ones, and the sad ones, the planned ones and those that arose unexpectedly, those that came early in life and those that happened yesterday. Your self-inventory reveals your strong suit—what you did best, what you liked to read—that you were an opera fan or enjoyed art museums. This inventory notes that you watched *Nova* on television, clicked occasionally on the History Channel, worked with your hands, tried new recipes and what newspaper ads captured your attention. The inventory also brought to the surface of your mind those special people you once admired and respected, as well as the sport you loved best along with your favorite hero.

"This is your life," as Ralph Edward used to say on the television show of the same name. From this large and lengthy pool of memories and forgotten experiences is the game plan to suggest your legacy. What counted in the past that will set up the plays that will change the score board?

Running through these life experiences can expose and identify your embedded passion or your purpose. Some may even describe it as 'my calling.'

Many people prefer not to think of their passion or purpose as a calling, because they associate the term with religion. But if you sincerely believe that you have a purpose in this life that is uniquely yours, you will understand that the idea of 'calling' is a natural, spiritual component of your inner being. When you accept the idea of your 'calling,' you will discover an immense power that sustains you in the process of attaining it.

In the mail today came a notice from a friend in New York. William J. Flynn had just arrived back in the States from Ireland after receiving a Doctor of Law *honoris causa* from the University of Ulster in Belfast, Ireland. Bill is 88 years old.

After Bill retired as CEO and Chairman of the Board of Mutual of America in New York City, he joined the Americans for a New Irish Agenda because of his deep roots in the Irish tradition. As a key figure within a United States contingency, Bill worked tirelessly to broker the first Irish Republican Army ceasefire that perpetrated the loyalist party ceasefire that followed soon after. The Irish President, Mary McAleese, described Bill's contribution to peace as "simply immense." Martin McGuinness, Northern Ireland's Deputy First Minister, declared him "one of the heroes of the peace process."

In presenting the degree to Bill, University of Ulster Vice Chancellor Brandon Hamber pointed out that Bill is "a man of vision who paid heed to his inner calling to make a difference in the world and in the land of his forefathers particularly. His life tells an extraordinary story. He has excelled in business and as a peacemaker."

This is the power of one man, who believed that his age was not a deterrent and his cause was right, and most of all, believed he was fulfilling his God-directed destiny.

THE FOURTH QUARTER

Principles of the Game:

The Seven Story Mountain by Thomas Merton

After taking an inventory of our life, let us take a look at what a Trappist monk discovered about his. Thomas Merton wrote and lived most of his life as a divided person. He lived with one foot in the secular world, the other in the spiritual. From his early life, he wrote that there was a noticeable disparity in his life's direction from the time of his baptism. "I don't think there was much power in the waters of the baptism…to untwist the warping of my essential freedom, or lose me from the devils that hung like vampires on my soul." These words signaled the beginning of the personal journey of a man who loved and thrived in a modern world before finally surrendering to the austerity and loneliness of a cloistered monastery.

In the last year of his life, Thomas Merton had a spiritual awakening after experiencing an encounter with God. He saw, for the first time, what God saw in him and in all human beings. "That everything visible has a hidden wholeness." Surprised at this insight, Merton described the experience as 'seeing,' and concluded that each individual has within him a particular 'hidden wholeness' that is only revealed in the presence of God.

That 'hidden wholeness' disclosed to Merton is the ribbon on the package of God's design for us. Scripture tells us, over and over again, that we are here for a purpose, not our own purpose, but God's purpose, and our hidden wholeness is achieved when we fulfill that purpose. Accepting that premise, we realize what we have been looking for it all our lives, and the response to it is our personal destiny.

WOW! What a Fourth Quarter breakthrough!

Our main concern now is to see this 'hidden wholeness,' within us as Merton did. To 'see' with an inner vision, perhaps for the first time, how God has, with great care and deliberation, directed our lives in the past, and now with this new insight, will guide and direct us in the future.

That's right. Direct our future. We are now in our fourth quarter. We are retired. Yet, we are possibly the most educated, the most experienced, and the most creative generation in history. There is no backing away from finishing the game or as Merton might want to say, fulfilling the 'whole.' To deny this is to deny all we have learned and all we have been given in preparation of this great hour.

Think about it. We are still alive for a purpose. Unfortunately, not everyone has been so blessed. For a man to die of a heart attack at forty-nine is sad beyond description, or for a young mother to develop breast cancer and be gone within six months is heartbreaking. But for those of us who have reached the fourth quarter, to live as if the game is finished is to deny our very reason for being.

This reason is your mission.

Searching now through your inventory of experiences, you are closer to 'seeing' your hidden wholeness. You have discovered the core values that helped you make decisions. You were reminded and confirmed as to your strengths and weaknesses. Your talents have been reinforced and you have learned from both good and bad experiences. Through the years you have faced situations with raw courage, tested your integrity and questioned your faithfulness. You have measured your patriotism and generosity and your spiritual life has either grown deeper or fallen through the cracks. You have survived battle wounds, occupational hazards, financial depressions, hospital stays, family feuds and dozens of children's ballgames and birthday parties. You have lived through an era of colossal change. This past century has gone from the horse and buggy to the moonwalk, from neighbors talking across the fence to cell phones and iPads, from a Judeo-Christian work ethic to a country of entitlements. From these involvements, documents and collective memories comes your unique history and this history tells you what has counted in your life and what will count going forward.

What counts in the past, predicts your calling for the future.

So what counts in your life—everything!

Listen for your name!

That's God calling.

From the Sideline

As one who is deep into the fourth quarter, I want to pose a new approach to the final years: the idea of 'forever beginning.' Taking the position that I am in my final days offends me. I reject the thought. Final is so…final. I am hitting the delete button on my computer and sending that word where all negative words should go. Because, for me, I will be 'forever beginning.' No matter what my driver's license says about my age, or that I am receiving Social Security, or that my blood pressure is slightly elevated, I will be forever beginning—something. Seeking that 'hidden wholeness' Merton mentioned coupled with the attitude of 'forever beginning,' I have the chance of viewing my future in a positive, self-actualizing way and finish my life with some measure of MAD (make a difference) accomplishment that changes the global imbalance, at least in my world.

My son once said, and his remark came as a surprise to me, that I am a driven woman. I had never considered myself driven. I thought about what he had said for days. He was right. I *am* driven. I am permanently locked in forward gear although at times the internal gear called 'forward' is often rusty, and I'm annoyed when the gear is slow in reacting. That is why I did what I am suggesting you do. I looked back into my past to find my hidden wholeness to explain who I am and guide me to where I should be going.

My inventory led me to a full blown memoir, which, when studied in depth, bared some innate traits that have lived within me. Now, when I ask myself what counts in my life, I can say first and foremost, it's 'freedom.'

My understanding of 'freedom' embraces several levels. I am free when external circumstances permit me to act as I desire. The democratic system of government has allowed me this freedom. As an American citizen I can come and go as I please as long as it does not interfere with another's freedom. I have the freedom of will, the power of choice, to make my own decisions; to co-create my future with God. To me, this free will is one of God's greatest gifts to human kind. To be able to decide, to choose, to prefer or desire for oneself is the most freeing gift of all. Without free will, artists cannot paint, musicians cannot compose, and politicians cannot give speeches. Without free will, a man cannot marry the woman he loves, or a woman cannot choose for her mate the man she desires.

As early as I can remember, I was operating as a free-wheeler breaking the proverbial parental shackles. When I was only three or four years old, I left home each evening to go with my neighbors to their dairy farm and help them prepare milk for the next day's delivery. In those days, dairy men delivered milk to their customer's back door. I had two jobs. One was to cap the milk bottles after the milk had been strained and poured into bottles. Then, I would ride in the front seat of the pickup, jump out and run the milk up to the customer's porch, leave the milk, and then pick up the empty bottles.

At that time, I never thought that I was either too young or too inexperienced to do the job. I only remember begging my neighbors to take me with them as often as they could. Where else, at that age, would I have had the opportunity to learn to milk a cow or cap a milk bottle? I was spreading my wings and having the time of my life and I was free to do so.

A couple of years later, my father, realizing I was a free spirit, built me a tree house in the back yard. The tree house was mine only. My brother was not allowed. I don't think he ever climbed that tree. But my father knew I needed a 'freedom' place of my own—a place to get away and just be. That tree house still lives, not only in reality, but in every word I think or write; for it was there that I read and began to write.

To say that I always used my freedom wisely is probably a rank overstatement. But, the misuse has never been strong enough to cancel or deter my need for freedom. I still have it.

Not long ago, I was attending a celebratory service in a cathedral in England. A young chaplain was preaching. It was Memorial Day. At the end of his sermon, he announced that he wanted to ask every civilian in the congregation only one question. The congregation waited riveted to their pews. The chaplain looked at us sharply and asked, "What have you done with your freedom?"

I ask myself that question almost daily. I live in a free country. As a woman, I can come and go at will, which is not true in other parts of the world. Until the 'politically correct' imperative invaded our country I could say or write anything I chose, and with discernment, I still do. But to answer the question of what I am doing with my freedom is simply to point directly to what you are doing right now—reading what I am writing. I am exercising the freedom to write the word 'God,' to discuss the idea of Christianity, and to speak boldly of my faith without fear of reprimand, or worse, either physical or verbal persecution.

Today, I am free to be, free to explore, free to venture out with new ideas and free to be myself in most situation. I also recognize that freedom goes beyond my personal need and becomes a right I wish for everyone. As an inalienable right, freedom is the basis of our national heritage, and should not be taken for granted but used wisely every day with appreciation and respect. What counts in my life as well is the value of learning. This includes, of course, reading and books, and this collective association causes me to say often, "I'll be a learner all my life."

This leads into another factor that defines my life—competition. I wish there was a softer word for competition, one less aggressive, but there isn't. Even though a more toned down word would suit me better, the truth is that I've been competitive all my life. From the time I played Pollyanna with my mother, to playing with marbles in grade school, debating in high school, and eventually running for Congress, I have played to win. It isn't that I have to win. It's that I have to play the game to win.

Gamesmanship, not the Las Vegas style that pits me against another person or a system or even myself, but life games compels me to continue regardless of the outcome. Today, I play Words with Friends, a digital game of Scrabble, with several people, most of whom beat me. Yes, that's right, they do. But I continue to play, win or lose, simply because I love the competition. Competition has always stimulated me to perform better, to work harder, and to finish on my feet. To be competitive has counted in my life for years. It still does.

However, as a life-long learner, my main frame of competition is intellectual. I *have* to know. The question came up the other day among the group as to who was the New Jersey congresswoman who smoked a pipe. I had known it previously, but it bothered me that I could not remember. Immediately, I whipped out my cell phone and looked her up. The answer was forthcoming and the discussion continued. I used to go to the library and delve deep into the catacombs of dusty books looking for answers. Now, I am delighted to be living in the internet era where most information is at one's fingertips.

My intellectual curiosity has taken me into previously unexplored places as well and I really relish the excursions. During our coffee meet-up, the discussion of competition arose when the group discussed whether or not our country was still competitive in the world. Lucy said she thought we had lost our competitive edge globally. Bob insisted we had not technically lost that. He said we were way ahead technologically even if the Chinese, Korean, and Japanese manufactured most of the new technology products. He cited a company by the name of Dapra, located in America, who began what we now know as the internet.

When asked if being competitive was a good or bad thing, Ralph commented correctly that the world of marketing is based on competition. Reed agreed and added that competition made products and services better. "If you are in business, you are by definition competitive."

Then, I asked who they thought was the most competitive person in the group. Their answer was instantly forthcoming. Jane was first with her quick answer—"You!" Bob agreed as did Roxie, so I took that honor, and I rest my case. Lucy and Frances took the silver and bronze medals.

I researched what being competitive really meant and with most definitions the word 'rival,' was cited, which to me indicated a warlike position. I view my competitiveness, not as combative, or as a tug-of-war, but more of a motivator. Competition motivates me, especially when an intellectual subject confronts me. Let an issue be brought up which I am totally unfamiliar, and I am the first to begin the quest for information on that subject. My competiveness (I believe) is grounded in 'wanting to know,' laced with a measure of curiosity.

Gratitude is also a personal, core principle for me. Often as I sit in a receptive mood, I am more conscious of being grateful than I am of being receptive. However, when I am grateful, I realize I am grateful for all that I have received even though what I receive settles in my right brain. My left brain must be dammed up, for I am technologically illiterate. Technically, I am a complete washout. To fix a television, my cell phone or my iPad sends me over the proverbial cliff. However, on the right brain side, I have had the good fortune to receive intriguing ideas, some that I have used while others lay waiting for attention. The other day when I was going through some of my old files, I found several fictional stories I had written years ago that I had completely forgotten. Also, in that pile were several manila folders marked 'ideas,' which I had discarded or allowed to go fallow. Activating those ideas would take me the rest of my life. Even unutilized, I am grateful to have had them.

These collective points of freedom, learning, competition, and gratitude help to define my mission. Together with the insight of my 'hidden wholeness,' I am acknowledging my purpose. And I continue to ask others like me:

> *So, what are you looking for, he said,*
> *From behind the curtain and under the bed?*
> *I don't know until I find it, she said.*
> *Is it from the friends you know or the books you've read?*
> *I don't know until I find it, she said.*
> *Stop looking, He said. Follow me instead.*
> *Oh, that's what I am trying to do, she said.*

Already in the Game

From my files comes a story of a person who has found his mission. His name is Jim Reid.

Ralph Miller wrote about Jim Reid in the *Dallas Morning News* this past year. It seems that Jim, who is well into his seventies, has started a new company called Momentum Texas. His business plan is simple, but profoundly innovative, useful, and proudly patriotic. His company mission is to help returning veterans become entrepreneurs.

Reid, with the aid of a grant from the Texas Workforce Commission, started his company when he learned that returning veterans had a higher unemployment and homeless rate than the

THE FOURTH QUARTER

overall population. Reid knew that 90 percent of the management knowledge gained by entrepreneurs comes from interaction with other entrepreneurs. Reid decided to join with the Veterans Business Assistance Program and set up a force of Dallas business men and women as mentor to these veterans.

The program quickly gained national attention and is now duplicated in many other cities around the country.

As a retired executive, Reid was not content with sitting at home in retirement. He marshaled his experiences as an entrepreneur into a worthy cause. A monetary value cannot be assigned to his project, because there is no way to fully calculate volunteerism. Reid's satisfaction is in watching his passion come to fruition in providing invaluable experiences for hundreds of young men and women of our armed forces returning home after battle. Reid had a clear purpose and a call to action.

Reid's legacy is many fold. When he posts that final score on the scoreboard, there will be thriving businesses around the country cheering him. Reid didn't sit around after his retirement. He found his passion—helping people. He concluded that he had been left on this earth for a reason, and he followed that reason to an ultimate and useful end. That's what counted for Jim Reid. I met them quite by chance. Their names are Pat and Harold Luck and they live in Toronto, Canada. Pat is a retired schoolteacher and Harold is retired from the real estate business. Now in their early seventies, they are teaching the international course of *Living a Healthy Life with Chronic Conditions*. This program was designed by Stanford University in California and is now taught internationally. The Lucks have been teaching this course so long that their students are now scattered throughout the country.

After teaching the course for several years, the Lucks were asked if they would like to instruct teachers. Today, they spend three days a week teaching teachers across Canada the methods espoused by the Living Healthy program. The program is now taught in 29 countries and in 12 different languages.

What an amazing and life-sustaining gift to give—that of health. The Lucks are Fourth Quarter people who saw a need, responded to it, and helped start a noble and worthy effort.

What counts with you? What should count is what you value, what you care about, and what you hold dear. What counts is what is sacred to you.

If what Jim Reid and Pat and Harold Luck are doing inspires you to do something, consider doing the following:

- Volunteering at the police station, hospital or church.

- Becoming email pals to a younger person.

- Clipping coupons and giving them to the local food bank.

- Planting a garden the entire neighborhood could enjoy.

CALL THE PLAY:
Joining the Game and Making it Your Passion

At another year I would not boggle. Except that when I jog, I joggle.
—*Ogden Nash*

Choices

We make a thousand choices a day, most of them trivial ones, like what to have for breakfast or should we turn down the air-conditioner or not. These are throw-away choices we pay little attention to because they are thoughtless, habitual, and routine.

But major choices, whether one is twenty or seventy, calls for our best intellectual efforts in order to avoid mistakes. Choices, such as lifestyle, career, life-mate and our future are made after a moral or ethical foundation is set in our formative years. These types of choices represent our value system which establishes judgment parameters and a guide or method for decision making.

One such method that helps in making decisions is the Wesleyan Quadrilateral that offers four benchmarks by which to test an idea and see what sticks. These four benchmarks are *reason*, *tradition*, *experience*, and *scripture*. By testing decisions against these four cardinal principles, one can find a satisfactory conclusion for any issue. When we ask ourselves: Is what I want to do reasonable, does it conform traditionally, has it been my experience that it works, and what does scripture say about this issue? This 'rule of thumb' system of decision-making, when thoroughly analyzed, gives us an assurance and comfort that our choice is a wise one. Often, all four aspects of the quadrilateral cannot be answered with complete satisfaction. If this is the case, it is best to go back and review the issue. It is never good to change the quadrilateral to conform to the issue. The risk is too great—far better to modify or change or even drop the issue entirely.

Flag Down

Consider the choice made by a couple who live on the West Coast. When they retired, they bought a lovely apartment overlooking the harbor at Oakland. Each day they get up, fix breakfast, then sit in their two favorite chairs facing the harbor and watch the boats come in and go out. They stay there until lunch time, have a bite of lunch, and then return to their chairs to watch and nap the afternoon away. At evening, the lights are on in the harbor and after dinner they sit again for an hour or two before going to bed. Their day is ended. Their life is ended as well.

Is their choice to do nothing reasonable? Is it in line with their traditional values? Have they experienced this before for themselves or others and found it satisfactory? Have they searched the scriptures before deciding to give up? Obviously, they have not.

But it didn't have to be this way. He was a banker with knowledge of finances and economics. Think what he could have accomplished in the years he spent in the rocking chair to help others understand their financial situation. He could have worked for a bank as their public relations person who counsels with new clients on how best to save, invest, and manager their incomes. He could have volunteered at a non-profit organization by keeping their financial records. He could have helped single mothers budget their income and learn how to stretch a dollar. A naval base was within blocks of his apartment. He could have volunteered to help the service personnel and spouses on how best to protect, invest, and save their incomes. The need for financial advice and counseling surrounded him, but it never crossed his mind. His wife could have worked one day a week at the naval base nursery or helped at the Post Exchange. Both of their expertise and personal capital was wasted while rocking in their chairs, satisfied that they deserved their leisure. They left the game early and never intend to return. What a shame. What a waste.

Principles of the Game:

The Choice is Always Yours (An Anthology)

In my library is a book that few people would claim ownership, but I consider it one of the most valuable books I have and refer to it often. A friend gave it to me, a friend whom I consider both academically and creatively minded, but that is not the only reason that makes this book special. To me, it is a wisdom book.

As an anthology of works from the earliest writings to the modern day, this book is more than about choice. It's about what your choices make of you. The introduction explains, "This anthology presents a mosaic of human insight. It has as its central theme a "Way" which all men seek, few find, few enter, and still fewer progressively follow, though it proffers the means by which man's most fundamental longing can be realized…. Deep in the psychic structure of every individual there is an urge for the kind of fulfillment which will yield meaning, joy and creativity."

In this most unusual book are thoughtful answers that pull us away from making destructive choices into making constructive ones. Believing that there is something of God in every person, or as I like to think, as the God within, this book works with various precepts to connect God with "the deep center," "the ground of the soul," "the inward voice," "the real self," "the inner vocation," or however you describe your ground of being. Whatever description you choose to relate to, every man and woman lives, admittedly or not, as if there is a Higher Power or Ultimate Reality in the universe. The degree to which this truth affects one is the degree to which a person make choices that connect him with that Higher Power.

One of the most comforting statements I know is 'the choice is always yours.' If this is true, then each of us can make that ultimate life-changing choice. And making that choice assures us that all subsequent choices will be right. That connective choice makes all the difference in making a difference. It's up to you. The choice is always yours.

Most of us have heard people remark from time to time, "I had no choice".... Well, yes, they did. The choices may appear impossibly bad, but you can always choose the best of the worst. Even if you choose not to choose, that, in itself, is a choice. The choice may be difficult, often considered impossible to make, but this book assures us that we always have a choice regardless of the situation, the circumstance, the people involved or the predicted outcome of a decision. To realize and acknowledge that we ALWAYS have a choice—regardless of the circumstance—adds an element of confidence and puts us in a different category of believers. No longer can we use, 'I didn't have a choice,' as an excuse or justification for our actions or lack of participation. All pretenses are gone, all alibis are weak, and all defenses are down. No apology needed and certainly no vindication for those who moan and groan about their inescapable dilemmas. Such freedom!

My coffee group had a field day with this topic. When first asked, "Are there situations in which we have no choice?" "Of course," exclaimed Lucy. "I agree," said Frances. It seemed everyone agreed. Roxie said, "The other day, a car almost hit me straight on as I was coming into the parking lot to park my car. I swung my car past my parking space to avoid being hit. I had no choice. I would have been creamed otherwise." Of course, Roxie made the right choice, but she did have a choice. She could have stopped and allowed the other car to hit her. She could have turned to the left and hit another car in the other lane, or she could have tried to wheel her car quickly into the parking space. But she said, "I had no choice."

Often the choices are not favorable or even wise. Sometimes, you simply have to make a dumb choice in order to relieve an awkward situation, but to say, "I didn't have a choice," is simply not true. When push comes to shove, there is a choice, be it ever so reluctantly made. Again, even if you decide not to choose, you are making a choice.

When a football game gets exciting, the quarterback has four options. He can lateral the ball to the tight end, he can pass the ball to the wide receiver, he can run with the ball himself, or he can knee the ball. These are the only four options he has to fulfill his purpose of moving the ball closer to the goal line. His purpose is clear; predefined and established as part of the rules of the game. He accepts his role and is committed to follow the 'rules of engagement' all the way to the goal line. One thing he cannot do—he cannot quit the game.

For those of us in the fourth quarter, what are our options?

We can pass the ball to another, then stand back and watch what happens. There is a feeling of relief when someone else is carrying the ball because we are no longer responsible. We are off the hook. But we are also sidelined, benched, and now relegated to being merely spectators.

A better option is to throw the ball to the wide receiver who is out there alone. If he catches the ball, he has a chance of going all the way. Or if we see a clear path, we can charge in and run with the ball through a massive amount of human barriers. What we can't do is leave the game…because we are alive for another day and we have a mission to do.

The Huddle

If you are fearful of carrying your mission alone and believe the heavy responsibility of winning is too much for one person, you need to rally a team of like-minded people who stimulate you, make you stronger, and help you follow through. Who are these people?

Look around you. Who thinks like you think? Who do you know who understands your plan and can help you strategize? Who makes suggestions and encourages you to follow through? Fourth Quarter people are everywhere. Look around you.

We are bunched together around a coffee table in a café; we are walking the mall in our best athletic shoes; or we are hovering around a guide at the Vatican listening as she describes the buildings. We are an elderly couple holding hands at the restaurant or searching for seats in a dark movie house. We are those old faces on motorcycles thinking we are as young as the gray panthers and we are those gray haired people climbing rocks around the Grand Canyon with cameras hanging from our necks. We are the adventuresome couple in our motorhome traveling the country and seeing most of it for the first time. We are the couple taking up the offering at the church, teaching Sunday school, or bringing dinner to a shut-in. Help is not far away. Whatever the purpose, we can help.

Carole Kanchier writes in her book, *Dare to Change Your Job…and Your Life*, that people don't lose their purpose; it just becomes hidden, buried beneath a lifetime of excuses, other priorities, and societal expectations. In fact, you are born with an innate purpose, and you can't change it. You can only give it a voice or deny it. It means that, even if you're seventy-five and have never before listened to your internal voice telling you to find your purpose, it's not too late. It's *never* too late.

For those of us in the Fourth Quarter, recognition of our God-given purpose provides us a greater degree of control over our days. We are more fruitfully engaged when we place a high priority on our calling. We wander less, we procrastinate less, we waste less time and we get things done. It is also true that having a purpose changes the way we behave. A commanding purpose changes our habits and our routines and shifts our actions from passive to active, because we have made a commitment that calls for perseverance and constant attention.

I was listening to Dennis Prager, a radio commentator, one afternoon when he was asked what is the greatest danger facing America today. His answer was simple but profound. He said, "A country cannot survive if it does not have a reason to survive. Our country was built upon an idea of 'In God we trust.' Our survival is a moral issue, and our greatest danger is losing our reason to survive, because we have not passed on to the next generation what America is all about." The same is true for individuals. We cannot survive if we do not have a reason to survive.

Prager must have been reading my notes, because I believe that as individuals, we must have a reason for living…or we become the living dead, and time will eventually consume us. When we think about it, there is no better reason for us as individuals to survival than to pass on to our children and grandchildren what it means to be an American. This reason may well be our purpose, a purpose with a moral component that changes others one at a time.

Purpose, by definition, implies activity. No one can tell another what his or her purpose is. I believe purpose is not lolling around the house watching television from morning until night for the rest of your life. Nor, heaven forbid, is it giving up on life because it is too much trouble to continue living otherwise. If this is your thinking, then reconsider. Consider the notion that there might be a reason that you are one of the privileged—that there is a clear reason you have been tapped to live in overtime. But, you ask, why me? Why have I been singled out to live into my seventies or eighties? The simple answer is obvious. You have been given a reason, a purpose, a calling, if you will—that completes God's plan for you to achieve.

Purpose is permanent and is never completely finished. Progress can be made. Milestones can be achieved. Landmarks may be established, but the work goes on. The game truly never ends. Scores are tallied along the way, and our time may run out, but the mission is still in motion.

Tactics and Strategies

Every endeavor, every business, every enterprise, and every person has a goal. Businesses want to manufacture tires to make money, the Red Cross wants to help people in emergency situations, enterprises seek to merge various businesses to form a coalition of companies, and individuals generally want, depending on their place in life, to marry, have a career, a family and a good retirement plan.

How these goals are accomplished depends upon the tactics and strategies designed specifically for them. Strategy defines the goal in specific objectives and how external forces relate or impinge upon your goal's success. It includes, for example, how other members of the family look upon your purpose and how it fits into to your schedule, how much time and money it will require. Strategic planning also consists of how best to present your plan to your family and friends, to set a budget and manage the time required.

Strategic planning also assesses the purpose in relationship to the goal itself. Is this my personal purpose or does my purpose involve others? Is my purpose a memoir or a social issue? Is my purpose vital to someone specific or to the society as a whole? Is my purpose limited or can it expand, and if it can expand, who will continue the plan? Strategic planning is a mental exercise done before any action can be performed successfully.

Tactics, on the other hand, is the physical exercise. What are the internal forces at work? What are the tools needed for implementation? When to begin and what comes first, second, and third? What other resources are required and how best to manage the budget? As someone said, "Strategy is doing the right thing; tactics is doing the thing right."

If this seems too formal for your purpose, break it down by all means. It is exactly what your mind will entertain as you entertain your purpose. Regardless whether you write down your particular strategy or not, you are thinking strategically on how best to obtain your goal. Whether you are consciously outlining your tactics in a step-by-step fashion or not, your mind is ahead of you clicking off the when, where, and how points of implementation. Your experience is surfacing; your personal skills are coming to the front and you are beginning to see the goal line. Your goal is already in your head and your heart. You have made your choice and your choice will now guide you. You can do this. You have mentally strategized a hundred times over.

In a Sunday morning edition of the *Dallas Morning News*, columnist Cheryl Hall wrote an article about an interview of Dallas notable, T. Boone Pickens. Boone was being interviewed by Sandi Chapman, the founder and chief director of the Center for Brain Health. "Boone is the poster child for brain health. He never stopped pushing the limits of his brain," said Chapman. Boone responded, "Last May I turned 84. I don't want to grow old and feel bad, either physically or mentally. That's why I exercise my body and my brain every day. When I was writing my last book, *The First Billion is the Hardest*, one of my guys suggested we go with a different title, *Living in the Fourth Quarter*. I told them I wouldn't know, because I am not there yet."

Chapman answers, "You're never too young and you're never too old to strengthen your brain's performance. Twenty-year olds aren't achieving their potential. Forty-year olds are letting their brains decline. Eighty-year olds go on automatic pilot instead of pushing their brains to keep achieving." When it comes to the future for Boone Pickens he has a regimen to keep him fit as a fiddle.

Boone says, "I still work out with a trainer most mornings at 6:30 before heading for the office. That's physical exercise but there's also a mental aspect to this. You have to stay involved and active. I've had too many friends who retire, spend too much time doing nothing, and they are gone before you know it. When I retire, it's going to be in a box. I have a lot left to do, and I'm capable of doing it. Remember, I didn't make my first billion until after I turned 70."

From the Sideline

My mission is called the Divine Afflatus.

From the time I was twelve I have been on a spiritual journey that has been more like a march or a campaign than a quest. I didn't need to find God, He found me. He found me as a child, as a teenager, as a young wife, as a mother, and now as a senior citizen, He is still finding me where He put me, sitting in front of a computer.

The day Pearl Harbor was bombed, I went to church alone. My parents never went. We were living in Louisville, Kentucky, and that day I had taken a city bus to a Christian Church about four or five miles away. I attended both Sunday school and Church and then took the bus home. That was many years ago. I am sorry I do not remember the minister's name or his sermon. I only remember his commission at the end of the service, after the benediction, standing at the back of the sanctuary and before the bells chimed, he quietly suggested,

> *'Er you go without these walls,*
> *Leave here your sorrows and cares.*
> *And in their stead, take faith and hope and love,*
> *These three, for they are thine.*

And then, within thy breast, great living altars raise
That you may meet him here, and then live with
Him at last forever more.

These words come to me today as vividly as they did more than seventy years ago. They affected me spiritually then and they still touch me now.

While living in Louisville, I had my first encounter with God. I was lying on my bed with my head at the foot of the bed looking through the upper window in my room at the sky. I don't recall the discussion held between God and myself, but I do remember having some kind of private understanding that He was God and I was the one to whom He was talking. God recognized me and I felt his presence, as simply, but as profoundly as a theological dissertation. Either I had been chosen, or I chose. Either way, I was committed. I told no one. There was no need. I was twelve years old.

Already in the Game

Their names are John and Colleen McKemie. They live in Sun City West in Arizona, a community of thirty thousand people. Both are retired. Now, John spends his days at an elementary school as a teacher's aide while Coleen spends her days at the local library as a volunteer. Recently, when John underwent heart surgery an avalanche of get-well cards flooded his hospital room. He sent some of them to me. Here are examples of notes from his second grade students, exactly as written:

1. Dear Mr. McKemie, You're a very nice old man you give hope to the second grade. Love, Gabriel.

2. I hope you get well soon McKemie we love you as much as Mrs. Collins and thanks for helping. Ian

3. Dear Mr. McKemie, we miss you. How are you? Did you have a

wonderful Christmas? How are you doing? You're the best person in the whole world. From Kaitlin

4. Hi Mr. McKemie, you are a very good man and thank you for all you did for us to make us happy. I rely like the book you got for me. Diego.

To add to their volunteer work, the McKemies make Christmas a special time for many in their community. John and Colleen become Mr. and Mrs. Santa on Christmas Eve. Dressed in full costume, they visit as many homes as possible that appear to be having a party. They may or may not know the people but they simply stop at each house, pop in briefly and wish everyone a Merry Christmas.

How memorable is that? John and Coleen are living out their retirement years with a distinct purpose…one that delights all who know them.

If what John and Coleen are doing inspires you, think about:

- Volunteering to help in Vacation Bible School.

- Painting a mural or clean up a local park.

- Building park benches.

- Establishing a safe walk to school events.

FATE or DESTINY:
Playing the Whole Field

The first forty years of life give us the text; the next thirty supply the commentary on it. —Arthur Schopenhauer

Destiny

I asked my coffee group the other day if there was a difference in fate and destiny. There was an immediate lull. I quipped, "Well, that went over big." Each said that they were thinking, but eventually, Bob said, "There's the manifest destiny that our country put forward years ago." Everyone was interested in what 'manifest destiny' was. Bob elaborated. "Manifest Destiny is the belief that the United States was destined to expand across the continent. The concept was born out of a sense of mission to redeem the Old World into a new heaven on earth." In other words, America was ordained by God to expand across the continent, and this belief provided the impetus to acquire all the land possible from Louisiana and Mexico and the British Empire, which it did.

History lesson aside, I asked my question again and the discussion went on. Frances didn't see any difference in fate or destiny, neither did Lucy or Roxie, but Bob commented that he thought fate had a more negative connotation than destiny, which is exactly true. Fate can be thought of as an accident or when a tornado touches ground, but destiny is believed to be designed by God, especially for individuals. Those of us who are survivors into the senior citizen category should not rely upon fate to guide us; we should rely upon our destiny. We see destiny as a fulfilling event, preplanned and ordained by God. But not everyone chooses to follow his or her destiny.

"Well, it was fate. That's all." A lament we've heard all our lives. When something bad happens, we have no other explanation for it, so we attribute it to fate. Fate is the culprit and the culprit is always bad news. Fate is generally looked upon as something normal human beings cannot do anything about. It is prescribed or fixed as an undisputable and irreversible law of nature and is always inevitable.

Destiny, on the other hand, is determined when individuals accept and make the choice to follow their destiny. Perceived as spiritually-led guidance, destiny is considered providential and consequently, positive and flexible. To follow one's destiny is to follow the path that God has predetermined. It is therefore spiritual rather than circumstantial. Destiny is universal, no one is left out. Again, destiny requires individual awareness and acceptance.

Principles of the Game:
The Soul's Code: A Search of Character and Calling by James Hillman

If you are a Presbyterian, you will understand fully the philosophical concept of psychiatrist Dr. James Hillman.

Dr. Hillman espouses 'The Acorn Theory,' which contends that each person bears a uniqueness that is destined to be what it is created to be, like an acorn that is genetically predesigned to become an oak tree. An acorn can never become an aspen or an elm tree. The acorn can only become an oak tree. Hillman believes that we are also predesigned with a genetic code that we cannot escape, change, or impede. We are who we are because of how God created us.

Hillman further explains, "The soul of each of us is given a unique *daimon* (spirit) before we are born, and it has selected an image or pattern by which we live on earth. This soul-companion, the *daimon*, guides us but often in the process of arrival we forget how we are created and believe we come empty into the world. But the *daimon* remembers. The spirit remembers our particular image and pattern, and in time it becomes the carrier of your destiny."

Hillman interprets this to mean we each have a calling. "That calling may be postponed, avoided, or intermittently missed, but eventually it will work itself out. It will make its claim. The *daimon* does not go away."

For some of us, this calling comes early in life and is clear. For others, this calling is still dormant and ambivalent. The danger we face is the likelihood that we stay so busy we forget or neglect or even ignore our calling. We allow our calling to seep away, like holes in a leaking vessel, until it has little strength to ever become active. But as Hillman says, the *daimon* does not disappear. It waits to be recognized.

Flag Down

I have witnessed this neglect of the creative spirit in the life of a retired friend. For over forty years he was a music professor at a university. Hundreds of students learned the value and beauty of music from this remarkably talented man. The music building was named for him when he retired. Now he lives alone tottering around his little bungalow, as he calls it, lonely and seemingly waiting to die. He tells me he is not waiting to die, he is busy all day. His 'all day' busyness consists of sitting in his chair listening to classical music. He says, "I'm thinking all the time."

One might question his mental activity as doing nothing but

reminiscing, and you would be right. To be fair, thinking is often one of the hardest jobs we can do, and thinking with a purpose, either to solve a problem or brainstorm a new idea, is even harder. But idle thinking is self-indulging. If he was truly giving his thoughts wings, he might activate the thoughts, cultivate them, put them into practice and pass them along to others. This friend, who was only busy in his head, could utilize his vast skills and experience by passing along what he knows to younger professors now teaching at the university. He could call them together once a month at his 'little bungalow' for an evening of discussion. What young professor, in his early years of teaching, would not welcome the attention and lessons from such a gifted and honored professor?

This thought never occurred to him. It never will. He died this morning.

From the Sideline

My purpose is a mind thing. In the Old Testament a statement says, "You shall love the Lord, your God with all your heart, soul and strength." The New Testament says "You shall love the Lord Your God with all your MIND, heart, soul and strength." I am a New Testament person. I believe that God made me mentally capable of deciding for myself. As the world changes so does my directives from God. I am to use my brain to listen, solve problems, clean up the mess in the house, initiate and complete a project or simply sit in solitude. My main job is to establish a connection, my mind with the mind of God.

As I mentioned, I am not a routine person. I don't want a daily schedule. As a free spirit, I want to be available to be or to do as unexpected events demand. I want to catch an idea on the fly or find a new friend in an unlikely place or hear music of the spheres from new and strange settings. I want to be available when someone asks me a favor. Like the other day, when I was sitting at the breakfast table in my pajamas early in the morning, a rapid knock came from outside my window. A neighbor was calling me in desperation. "You have to take me to the emergency room." I jumped up, shoved on a pair of jeans, put on my shoes and grabbed the car keys and was off taking this friend to the emergency room at the hospital.

Think about it. I was sitting quietly, reading the paper when my neighbor called. What would she have done had I not been sitting where she could see me? It was no coincidence. I was sitting there for a reason. She needed me. And she needed me at that moment.

I would not trade that affirmation of my reason for being for anything in the world.

Already in the Game

Yesterday, I received a telephone call from my friend Omar Harvey. He wanted to know if he should write a book about his former business connections. I asked if he felt like he should. And he answered. "Funny, you should ask, for that is exactly what I feel. I should do this."

Omar will be 92 on his next birthday. When he called, he was on his way to the barber shop and then out to dinner. I recited the acorn theory to him and suggested that he perhaps was predestined to write his book. I could feel him smile over the phone. "Thanks," he said and we hung up our phones. I will tell you, without a doubt, he will write that book. Whether he considers writing the book his destiny or his final contribution to the world is not for me to say. But the results will be an immeasurable value to a host of people who worked with him in his former company and to a larger host of employees there today.

Is Omar's nudge to write this book a 'calling,' a 'purpose,' or the '*daimon*'? Is it that 'still small voice' or that 'gnawing itch?' Is it a dormant hidden wholeness that is now demanding to be released?

No one can write that particular story but Omar. If the story is to be written, he knows that he is the one to do it. Knowing Omar, he will tell you, up front, it's a CALLING.

There is nothing more fascinating, as well as obligating than a true 'calling.' The way I look at it, I cherish the idea of a 'calling' because if God asks me to do something, He is not going to leave me without the means to get it done.

###

One Sunday morning while having breakfast at a restaurant, my friend Rod Keitz came up to me and said, "Dede, let's do a children's book."

"Rod," I answered, "I've never written a children's book. What kind were you thinking about?"

"Oh, maybe something about 'fish.'"

I knew less about fish than I did about writing for children, but I went home and considered his idea. Fish did not say anything to me, but I thought on. The next Sunday we met again for breakfast. I said, "Rod, what about computers? Could we do a young children's picture book about computers?" Rod loved the idea and within two weeks, *Henry the Hard Drive* was born.

Rod has been retired for over twenty years as one of the premier graphic artists in Dallas. When he retired, he put away his art board, his magic markers, his computer software program, and openly said, 'I'll never draw again. Art is over for me.' And he stuck to his pronouncement. Now, as Rod is approaching 80, he has dusted off his easel, booted up his computer art program, and brought his talent back onto the field. *Henry the Hard Drive and His Friends* was published this fall; the first three books in a series of eight.

CALL TIME:
Recognizing the Sense of Urgency

Age is like the newest version of software—it has a bunch of great new features but you lost all the cool features the original version had.
—Carrie Latet

It's About Time

MAD (Make a Difference) Fourth Quarter people are limited. Our time-outs are in single digits. As each day passes, we become more sharply aware that time now is a diminishing asset, and like everything else that hits us at this age, we must deal with it at the scrimmage line.

As long as we have lived with time, time still eludes our understanding. Time is pervasive and omnipresent, resisting our efforts to isolate or define it, suggesting that time is outside ourselves, something which passes, something we spend or serve or kill, something which, though admittedly a part of the natural order, runs a course all its own without our control or assistance. We cannot order time to speed up or slow down. We can't overrule time or demand it to change. We don't own or govern time. Its process is not in our hands, and we don't know how much or how little is left until our lease expires. At our age, all we can do is use time to a greater advantage. Like the writer Letty Progreton, says, "Age is a number and mine is unlisted."

That fact forces us to consider time as critical. If we are not careful, time will eat away our minutes and days like termites eating away the infrastructure of our homes until our house is completely destroyed. Without our input or final vote. time, on its own, has elected and enacted its irrevocable rules.

Therefore, we must not be consumed by time's greedy inroads or miss the opportunity to complete our destiny.

Instead, we must consider time not as a robber, but as a benefactor—a giver of gifts just at the right time. We might not understand time, but we should not resent it. We should make friends with it and use what time we have left wisely.

Years ago, I spoke to a group of senior citizens on the subject 'It's About Time.' I did not dwell on the physics of time and space as a scientist might have done, but I warned my audience of the many decisions they would have to make as they faced their declining years. Where should they live, with whom should they live, and what financial resource would be required to go the distance?

My speech was part of a seminar sponsored by the Senior Citizens of Greater Dallas. The seminar dealt with all aspects of living past age 65, including financial, emotional, and the physical considerations of everyday life. Several hundred people were in attendance, and some of them, mostly women, told me that many people often go through life totally uneducated, ill-prepared and ill-equipped with the survival tools necessary to cope effectively when they are left alone. For many of the attendees, they had not given advanced age a thought until they found themselves slap dab in the middle of it, and had to face it head on without preparation.

That leads us to understanding the difference between quality and quantity time. Our quantity time is uncertain, but the quality of time we can determine. The term 'quality time' has been with us since the early seventies, when it was thought that parents were not spending enough time with their children, especially if both parents worked. The term meant time dedicated exclusively to a certain person, mainly a child. For us, taking the same definition, quality time must be dedicated to a special, concentrated, and deliberate effort to make a difference. Time is a gift, but dedicated, quality time holds a battery of gifts that reinvent and evolve over and over again.

If we look at our remaining days as a gift, we immediately view life in a new way. And when we view something in a new way, new meaning takes shape. Time can no longer be ignored with indifference or complacency. Time has innate power and perpetual motion; within its sphere of influence is action and reaction. Time possesses heart and courage; compassion and dedication. Time, used creatively, gives us encouragement and insight, inspiration, and spontaneity.

These are the surprise gifts of time that are not calculated in minutes, months, or days, but recognized as a companion to the fulfillment of our mission.

The extent to which we perceive time as a positive, and not a negative variable, bears greatly on our ability to keep going. The extent to which we feel the urgency of the clock ticking bears heavily on our behavior, adding pressure to make a difference now rather than in the future. One thing is for sure, though. We are knee-deep in the fourth quarter and our time in the game is ticking away.

The impediments, restraints or barriers that have held us back, due to previous commitments and earlier decisions, are now no longer relevant. We are retired and time cannot wait.

Before retirement, we believed that our busyness defined our value to the company where we worked. It was company time and time management meant squeezing as much activity as possible into the shortest amount of time possible in a frenetic attempt to finish and finish well. Our time belonged to the company. Our identity was derived from the company. The company supported us and in a very real sense, owned our minds and our energy.

Time management for MAD Fourth Quarter people is defined differently. It means adjusting the time we've pruned from chauffeuring, professional meetings, and daily grocery-buying into a less frenetic state. Our activity in the morning is no longer quickly grabbing a piece of toast and heading out of the door at 7 a.m. into a world of traffic. We can reset the action clock to our own speed and shift our priorities to activities that reduce our blood pressure, stabilize our heart rate, and calm our nerves.

And that's as good as it gets.

Principles of the Game:

A Sense of Urgency by John P. Kotter

John P. Kotter wrote the best book I know explaining the sense of urgency. He says the sense of urgency means something of 'pressing importance.' "When people have a true sense of urgency, they think that action on critical issues is needed *now*, not eventually when it fits easily into a schedule."

To me, a sense of urgency equates to an imperative, an obligation that demands attention. This imperative drives me to my desk chair and compels me to buckle my seatbelt. I wondered if my coffee group friends are affected in the same way?

Their responses to my question about their sense of urgency surprised me. I thought most of them might think as I do, but that was not the case. When I asked straight out if anyone felt a sense of urgency due to age and time constraints about what they were hoping to do in the future, Frances said immediately. "I feel nothing at all." Several nodded in agreement. When I queried

THE FOURTH QUARTER

further about what they felt they should be doing in their last years, I was shocked that most of them said, "Nothing." They are a highly educated group and I was disappointed, but then I thought, these friends are the perfect audience for this book. They have the most to give and their contributions would be invaluable to others. What were they thinking?

Their responses also indicated to me the true enemy of aging—complacency, the antithesis of a sense of urgency. Those who felt no sense of urgency seemed to be satisfied with the status quo and perhaps considered their professional years adequate.

But consider the fact that both a sense of urgency and complacency have innate powers. One stimulates, motivates, and renews itself every day. The other renders one useless and non-productive. In a very real sense, the two are at war with each other and unfortunately some people opt to take the easy, less demanding alternative and in the process lose out.

The one indisputable companion that accompanies a sense of urgency is the sense of being fully alive. Knowing that whatever is created by this sense of urgency is supremely important.

I, therefore, agree with Kotter's summary: "At the very beginning of any effort to make changes of any magnitude, if a sense of urgency is not high enough and complacency is not low enough, everything else becomes so much more difficult."

The other obvious enemy of a sense of urgency is 'comfort.' I'm talking about the "I don't give a damn" people who are content to lounge around in their comfort zones. They have found the comfortable temperature, the comfortable friends, the comfortable diet, and the comfortable routine and they don't want to be shaken out of their comfort zone. Their productive days are over, and they celebrate by frittering away irretrievable time.

Complacency or comfort is the enemy, not time. If we are not cautious, complacency or comfort will take over and cancel the urgency and potency of time. When the inner voice says, 'It's good enough,' or 'Its close enough,' complacency cancels our resolve and causes counter-productive inertia. With that attitude, accomplishing anything worthy is almost impossible. The seduction of complacency's power always vies for our attention. Precious little is required of us and giving into the rocking chair syndrome is taking the lazy way. But complacency is often detrimental to our physical health and frequently devastating to our mental health. The complacency of self-satisfaction is a crippling disease that slips up on us unaware.

For Fourth Quarter people, the sense of urgency may first show up only as a feeling or a psychological nudge, or even a wish, or it may be, like Frances said, "Nothing at all." She does not feel that time is rushing her or pushing her. She is happy to allow each day to come and go without thinking of what might be.

Janet, on the other hand, feels that urgency. She said she realizes she must be doing what she should be doing, because she senses keenly her own mortality. Both she and I look upon a sense of urgency as invaluable, as a directive and a confirmation of what we are about. Janet is probably the youngest member of our coffee group, and she comes every morning riddled with physical pain. Yet, she is the one who offers to repair anyone's cranky computer, to pitch in and help any of us move, or to give counsel on investments. She is totally forward looking. Her conscious need to keep moving forward solidifies her resolve to make a difference. This plaguing feeling of fleeting time helps Janet reinforce her independent determination to make a difference.

I have a sense of urgency—big time. As a writer, I have several book ideas that I wish to put on paper, but wonder if I'll have the time or energy to complete any of them. However, I feel the urgency to try.

Janet and I share this feeling from many levels. If there is a new technological toy coming out, our names are on the list to receive it hot off the production line. We got our cell phones before any of the others in the group. We got our iPhones and right on the heels, we got a Kindle and a Nook. We're waiting now for the upgrade of the iPad and the new iPhone 5.

This sense of urgency is built into my DNA like an obligation that demands attention with a high degree of insistence piled on top. It's one of those things that you cannot outgrow or use up.

In this regard, a sense of urgency is invaluable. There is no substitute for getting things done. If the boss is expecting a business proposal tomorrow, there is a sense of urgency to finish the project. If guests are coming for dinner on Friday night, there is a sense of urgency to prepare the house. Or if an essay is due on Friday and this is Thursday, there is an acute sense of urgency to finish. This sense of urgency then is the power machine that activates and often changes our behavior, making it one of the most beneficial motivators of all.

Think of the times you were part of a crisis situation and felt a sense of urgency. Years ago, when I was very young, I ran upon a terrible accident. It happened mere seconds before I drove up. It was about ten o'clock at night, and it was dark and difficult to see exactly what had happened. I got out of my car, rushed to the scene and noticed four cars jammed up in the middle of a four-way intersection. People were hurt. Since this was long before cell phones, I yelled to my friends in my car to go for help; call the police and an ambulance. I flew back to see what I could do physically to help.

This was a crisis. Action was important and there was an imperative to do something immediately. The urgency of the situation motivated my behavior. My adrenalin was flowing and I realized I was the one in charge. Assessing the situation in seconds rather than minutes, I checked for those either injured or dead. I calmed the hysterical victims the best I could and tried to organize those who soon came to help.

This extreme case illustrated the power that comes with the feeling of urgency. In these cases, one often acts in ways one could not or would not do under lesser circumstances. I was certainly doing things I was neither trained to do nor thought I could do. This accident demanded an urgent response from whoever happened to appear on the scene.

Also, I feel the sense of urgency now that I am a MAD Fourth Quarter person. I would like to go to Portugal and Spain before I can no longer travel. I would like to finish a major novel before I can no longer type. And I hope I have enough time to see the broader world in better shape politically. All this requires time.

So our attitude, toward the time we have left, is important. Time is not our enemy even though it has us by the short hairs. With dedication, commitment, and persistence, time still yields dividends, especially if we treat the clock with respect, hospitality and honesty.

The difference in looking at time now versus when we were twenty or thirty years old is that the urgency is paramount. We know we must plunge ahead if we are to score and leave this world better than when we arrived. This sense of urgency is joined with a renewed sense of being alive and whatever is created vibrates with importance.

From the Sideline

I look at my sense of urgency on a philosophical level. I believe I do not have the right to disappoint. The scriptural admonition, 'To whom much is given much is expected' haunts me constantly. I have been blessed, throughout my life, beyond the universal standards of living. And most of my blessings are the result of what others have done for me, not what I have done. I have had very little to do with my state of being at the present time. It is undeserved grace. There is simply no other explanation. As someone said, this makes me a walking arrangement of the Hallelujah Chorus.

To disappoint God, my friends, my family, and above all, myself, is totally unacceptable. I know God expects me to use the gifts given to me. My family has expectations of me, and I am awash with a sense of urgency to satisfy this compelling desire to make a difference.

Two of my favorite books are: *Fifty Who Made the Difference*, published by Esquire Magazine and Harold Evan's book, *They Made America*. Each book chronicles the lives of Americans who have etched their contributions permanently into our country's culture stone. I will never be one of those people and my small efforts will never be cast in stone, but I will never excuse myself for not trying to do what I know I should do. I will always be a person 'under construction.'

On a more practical level, this sense of urgency keeps me focused. It also makes me careful while at the same time frees me to risk whatever is needed to further my projects. I can't afford to waste time any more that I can afford to feel self-satisfied with what I do. So often I resemble the parable about the man who said he would do something, but did not, and the man who said he wouldn't do something, but did. As much as I might resist, I am that person who will quickly says, "No, I am not going to do that," and then end up doing it. A sense of urgency doesn't allow me to get by with saying no. Some might call this my conscience speaking, and that has a part, but when I end up doing what I said I would not, I do it immediately. There is an urgency to correct my mistake, to recover and move on. If I do, then I can release the assignment and the motivation as well as the guilt associated with my not complying in the first place.

Then, selfishly, I have to confess, the sense of urgency gives me an out. I use urgency when I need to justify saying 'no.' I can, very easily, and without one whit of remorse, tell someone that I am sorry, but I simply do not have the time to go to lunch with them, or shop at the mall or take a weekend excursion.
Finally, I can say that for me this sense of urgency will not go away. Like fleas on a dog, this sense of urgency causes me to itch

every day of my life. I live with it, scratch it when needed, or treat it every day.

Already in the Game

My friend, Ned Startzel, best known as the Rotary Singer, read one day in the newspaper about a man named Mark Carroll who wanted to start a senior's follies reminiscent of the Ziegfeld Follies but featuring the community's most talented seniors. Ned never considered his own age before contacting Carroll to say, "Include me in."

Ned spent hours recruiting and rehearsing seniors in song and dance routines.

Within weeks, the Spectacular Seniors Follies was born, and for three years, Startzel, a very personable man in his eighties, and his friends performed on stage to full houses in concert halls all over north Texas. Mark Carroll, the man Startzel contacted and the producer of the show, said, "From everyone involved in the production to everyone who enjoys the show, it proves that life in the golden years is just as exciting as it ever was. It transformed lives."

Ned Startzel didn't consider the element of time either. He didn't ask himself if he had enough days or months or years to become a part of the Seniors Follies. He simply dialed the telephone and the music began.

How cool is that?

###

Today Mike Snyder is in a wheelchair. For years he worked at the North Dallas Food Bank distributing food to the needy. Several months ago, he was in an accident leaving him permanently crippled. After two months in rehab, he was still unable to walk and could not even hold a cup of coffee. They told him he would spend the rest of his life in a wheelchair. But that didn't stop Mike from working at the Food Bank. Now, instead of doling out food, he has been made volume manager, keeping track of the food coming in and going out at the Food Bank. He tells his friends that on his bucket list (what he wants to do before he dies) is a visit to Tuscany to learn about wine.

When a friend heard about Mike's desire to go to Italy, he told him to get ready. Tuscany was in his future. Today the two men are touring Tuscany in a Jeep, learning about wine and the famous wine country. Both men are in their seventies.

If Ned or Mike's experience inspires you, you can consider:

- Volunteering at the Salvation Army store.

- Volunteering at the local library to re-shelve books.

- Driving the church bus to various functions.

- Offering to shop for groceries for a shut-in friend.

- Working as a receptionist at your church.

THE WIDE RECEIVER:
Opening Up to the Opportunities

The most pathetic person in the world is someone who has sight but no vision.
—Helen Keller

Out in the Open

We MAD American Fourth Quarter people have a lot going for us. Most of us are healthier than ever, have a better lifestyle than most people in the world, have enough financial resources to see us through to the end, and have not lost our sense of humor. We have amassed years of experience in a variety of disciplines and have voted for or against twelve or thirteen different presidents. We have watched the world change from rural to urban, from manufacturing to service, from homogeneity to diversity.

We have witnessed astronauts going to the moon and Navy Seals eliminating a known terrorist leader. We have survived at least three major and two lesser conflicts, a national depression, and the devastation of September 11th. We have enjoyed capitalistic growth, bought and sold stocks and bonds, and have owned at least two houses, a fishing boat, and two exercise bicycles. We have driven everything from a Model T to a Lexus, ridden everything from horses to ski mobiles and have traveled for pleasure and business across the globe. Best of all, some of us have participated in creating the greatest generation. As Ethel merman sang, 'Who could ask for anything more?'

But we are not done.

Dr. Paula Harden, an expert on generative people, garnered an impressive, cohesive list of intangible qualities from her research as a clinician and says that successful aging people who are maturing positively have the following attributes.

We have evolved a generous view of others and of the world, which includes maintaining a forgiving stance toward faults and inadequacies in ourselves and others.

We have a giving attitude toward ourselves and others. We give more financially than do most.

We form a caring and positive relationship with nature. We are concerned about the quality of the environment that will be passed on to future generations.

We are reflective and seek self-understanding.

We have had a pivotal event or events that led to transition or re-birth experiences. Everyone has such events, but generative people use them to grow and expand while non-generative people withdraw and blame others for their misfortunes.

We simplify our lives. Generative people take time to gain the insights needed to clear away clutter and confusion. We learn to set limits.

We have the courage to change both ourselves and conditions around us.

We describe ourselves as spiritual. We trust God or some Higher Power, and we trust the life process.

THE FOURTH QUARTER

We are sought out by other for counsel, wisdom, perspective, and creative insight.

We are committed to continue learning. We often spend considerable time learning on our own or attend a variety of workshops and classes.

We are clearly engaged in caring behavior toward ourselves and others.

We are involving healthier eating and exercising patterns.

We find laughter and tears coming easily and spontaneously.

We are hopeful people. We take our dreams seriously, and our lives demonstrate that some dreams do come true.

We have the courage to deal with our own mortality, making appropriate plans as needed.

We are also suited up for the game.

We are retirees with long careers in business, in education, in the health industry, in the arts, in the public and private sector and now we are wide open for opportunities to fill our remaining years with personal satisfaction, in order to make a lasting difference and complete our God-directed calling. As retirees, we have reevaluated our positions, shifted our attitudes, changed our lifestyle and negotiated for newer skill sets. Some of us are down the field and close to the goal line. Others like us are still at the line of scrimmage, waiting for the ball to snap.

That is why it is important to consider ourselves a wide receiver.

So who are the wide receivers?

Wide receivers are visionaries. We take the long view and open ourselves up for unimaginable possibilities. We view issues and subject matters from a distance with 360 degrees of insight. We have learned to think with sophistication due to our extensive reading and our wide range of experience. MAD Fourth Quarter wide receivers have a secret weapon—we have visions of what might be, what can be, what ought to be—because we are viewing life and life's solutions from a wider, longer perspective than younger people.

We are willing to consider new ideas and new solution paradigms. Ours is an enviable position.

In the Broadway musical 1776, there is a scene in which John Adams is trying to convince his fellow countrymen of the wisdom of independence. As he paced the floor of Independence Hall, he said, "Doesn't anybody see what I see?" At that point, only John Adams was envisioning a new America, free from British rule, autonomous and self-governing. To his credit, John Adams' vision was so clear and his passion so compelling that he convinced his fellow countrymen to his way of thinking. America is America today because one man stood up, with a cause larger than himself, stayed the course and won. John Adams was not only a man of vision; he was open and receptive to an idea that seemed ludicrous to some and implausible to others, but proved wise enough to create a new country.

Wide receivers, by definition, are always open. In football, the wide receiver positions himself at the far end of the offensive line, prepared to sprint forward into the open field as soon as the ball is snapped. He is the long pass catcher. He must be a fast runner, quick to adjust and willing to dive into the air to snare an overthrown pass. Agility and commitment are keys to his success. Big hands and long arms help.

Wide receivers cultivate the ability, as well as the habit, of receptivity. Now that we have the time to rethink and reevaluate many of our past notions and beliefs, we can spend time to formulate those thoughts into full evolution. For instance, most of us are hard-wired to certain ways of thinking. Take the adage, 'It is better to give than to receive.' We have been taught this adage from childhood and have taken this Jesus phrase as irrefutably and absolute. Doing this may have benched us from learning another essential but elemental lesson about being receptive.

Good receivers do not function well in traditionally structured, restrictive environments. We bristle under too much authority and too little freedom of thought and action. Good receivers question the hackneyed adages and admonitions, such as 'haste makes waste,' or 'a penny saved is a penny earned,' or 'it is better to give than to receive.' Some people adopt these ubiquitous lore-isms without question or further consideration. They believe them as they are, pattern their lives accordingly, and subsequently close out any suggestions of verification. That's the way it has always been, so why change?

Mature receivers say, "Let's take another look." Or, "Who says so? Or, "Why do we believe this?" We take the time and effort to re-examine the ordinary and the familiar and take a more maverick approach to traditional or commonly held notions in pursuit of truth.

Even as team players, mature receivers are self-directed. Being self-directed implies a healthy measure of self-confidence and self-assurance. We believe we have a stake in the future and some influence upon its direction. Like a wide receiver on a football team, we are goal setters and achievers, and have our eyes faced straight ahead. We don't look back. Self-directed wide receivers are starters with an intuitive sense of our abilities to start a project, be it a building or a company or a tree house.

Mature wide receivers avoid depression by the sheer impetus of curiosity about what could be. Aware of our goal, the score board and time, we know how to get there often by separating ourselves from the body of the team. If need be, we stand alone ready for the special moment to seize the opportunity.

Clichés are not unfamiliar to my coffee group. When I tossed this question, 'Is it better to give than to receive' they each had a ready answer. Reed said, "You give because it makes you feel good."

Roxie said, "You give because you see a need." Lucy remarked that every morning she thanks God for all she has been given and so naturally she would want to share. Everyone was quick to respond to the giving part.

Then I asked a question. "Is it possible to give something you have not first received?" They were slower to answer. Finally, Jane said, "We have all received more than we thought we ever would in material things." Roxie concurred. "We have more than any other people in the world."

"Yes," I said, "but back to the original question. So, is it better to give than to receive?"

"Of course, it is," was the universal conclusion. Everyone knows that.

Bob chimed in and added, "Maybe 'receiving and giving' are not separate actions. "Maybe they are two sides of the same coin." The discussion rolled on with more questions than quick answers, but we all concluded that whether better or not, it is a fact that we have learned to give better than we have learned to receive. My next question followed, "So then, aren't we all poor receivers?"

Jane remarked that receiving is often uncomfortable, "Like receiving a compliment. When someone says, 'I like your dress,' we generally slough off the remark by answering. 'Oh, this old thing, I've had it for years.'" Chuck, remembering his military days, said "It always embarrasses me when someone says I'm a hero. Listen, the heroes are the ones who didn't come back. I'm not a hero; I just did my job, so I shrug my shoulders as if what they said is not true."

Is this false humility, lack of proper receptivity or, to put it bluntly, rude? Both men and women are often self-conscious when paid a compliment. Clearly, this self-effacement means we have not learned nor have we had much practice in being a receiver. In most incidents, a simple 'thank you' would suffice.

When I was in graduate school, I took a course in psychology. At one particular session the instructor had us sit in a circle and randomly pointed to a young woman in the circle and told the rest of us to only tell this young woman positive things about herself. We began. I don't remember the exact words that were said, but compliments were immediately forthcoming. After about three or four had spoken, the young girl burst into tears and flew out of the classroom.

I waited only a few second, then excused myself, and went out to find her. I did not know the girl, but I wanted to comfort her if I could. She was sitting on the steps outside the building. I sat down beside her. She was still crying. When I asked if I could do anything, she said, "I couldn't take it. No one has ever complimented me like that."

What a great lesson in receptivity, as well as a poignant illustration on how hard it is to hear and receive compliments. She could not successfully accept compliments because she had no experience in receiving them. Criticism she could have taken better, at least to a point, but compliments brought out deep feelings of unworthiness and praise was too hard to accept.

The night I interviewed Bryan and Doneita Forrester, some special friends of mine, on the subject of receptivity we spent two hours engaged in nose-to-nose conversation about the subject. As the evening drew to a close I thanked them for meeting with me and allowing me to test this idea of receptivity on them. "Oh, it was our pleasure," Bryan said. "You honored us by asking."

"Oh," I said, "it's not that important," and immediately all three of us broke out in laughter. I did it to myself. I realized I still could not receive a compliment easily. The humility lesson was so firmly embedded in the psyche. However, this time for me, the humility lesson was learned and filed away.

Being receptive is a major, natural component of our human structure and part of our functioning system whether we are conscious of it or not. Our senses are all receptacles. Our eyes receive light, our ears sound, our noses smells and our mouths food. We receive constantly and unconsciously. We have perfected the physical part of being receptive, but have fallen short or neglected exposing ourselves to the emotional, spiritual and psychological aspects of receptivity.

Consequently, the scale is out of balance. Giving outweighs receiving. Seeking to correct that imbalance, we need to be proactive in our effort to properly receive, like an economist tests the imbalance between the classic equation of cause and effect, or supply and demand. For the truth is, there is simply no way we can give without first receiving, even though we have lived for years uncomfortable with the receiving portion. Thus receiving is undervalued and consequently, underdeveloped.

Since we are receptive creatures and our senses are constantly receiving light and sound, smells and taste, let's look at our receptivity in relationship to our physical make up.

Take the eye. The eye consists of many receptors called retinal rods and cones. The cones, for instance, are centered in an area called the fovea and receive and absorb either blue or green or yellow colors giving us Technicolor vision. By contrast, the rods, which are twenty times more numerous than the cones, accept the darkness filtering out the light, thus allowing us to see in the dark.

More specifically, when our eyes scan a room they catch certain objects; the cluttered desk, the lighted computer, the green drapes and the magazine on the table, the books on the shelves and the waste paper basket filled to the brim. Although the eye has the capacity of seeing everything, it does not. Not all the objects in a room reach the brain to register their presence. The brain quickly discriminates what the eyes see, leaving only what is wanted and leaving out what is unwanted or unnecessary. Eyes are selective receivers. If you are looking for a paper clip your eyes will search for it on the desk rather than on the green drapes. Since paper clip, are generally found on a desk, eyes do not bother to scan the entire room in search of them. The eyes pick and choose from a vast number of objects, colors and shapes in order to limit the intake by the brain. We selectively receive. And we do this as wide receives as well. We don't attempt to catch every ball, only those that are directed to us specifically.

Every step of the complicated process of seeing is made by one receptor passing the image or impression to the next receptor. And the eye, as well as the nose and ears are receivers that send messages to the brain which dutifully identifies and interprets the message.

The brain is even more complicated than the eye. Without going into a scientific explanation of how the mind works, let's simply review the data from the many years our minds have been receiving.

A baby is born—and immediately wrapped in a receiving blanket. No surprise there. Newborn babies are instantly and inherently receptive. In the very early stages of development, being receptive is the most natural thing babies do. They instinctive know how to receive milk, and soon they reach for their bottle. A baby's brain tells him, the bottle is important, vital to him. Not as flashy maybe as the wind mobile over his bed, yet the baby quickly discerns the bottle as necessary, comforting and satisfying. Toys follow in importance. However, a baby is totally unaware of the furniture in the room, the roast in the oven, the headlines in the newspaper or the bills in the mailbox. What is important and what is trivial to a baby changes as he grows.

As the years go by, the brain collects, retains, catalogs and archives data upon data. Our modern computers graphically illustrate this. I am putting words into a computer at this moment as I write. My words will stay there forever, unless the computer crashes or I perform an erase error. With a single punch of the 'save' key, words are stored permanently now with iCloud and Dropbox, the data is warehoused forever somewhere in a centralized storage bank. At present, my computer stores five of my completed books utilizing mega-bytes of storage and as marvelous as that is, the computer, on its own, can only bring back what I have stored there. The computer cannot invent, create, or have independent ideas. It does not speak for itself, cry or laugh. The computer cannot climb a mountain, sail a boat or bring forth a child. Yet, as a brain, my computer can mirror my words, receive my thoughts, accept my mistakes, and amass tangible data for me regardless of where I might be in the world. Like the brain, the computer is a huge receptacle—trained and programmed to return whatever has been received. With algorithms, it can now discern what is significant and what is trivial.

That's a brain job of our MAD Fourth Quarter wide receivers. From what has gone into our lives for six decades or more now can come back in remarkable, innovative and creative ways. All that is stored up in our brain cave can be booted up to suggest and clarify our purpose or mission. From what we have received through the years, we can reproduce in triplicate or in a different form, or with different meanings. We can use this data and these experiences, stored in our mental computer memory, for something that matters.

As clever as the computer is, an essential component will always remain out of the computer's range of capability. The computer cannot pray. Only human beings can pray. And I believe that the experience of prayer comes closer to balancing the giving/receiving equation than any other means available to us.

Brother Lawrence had the right idea. In his little book, *Practice the Presence*, he said, "The time of business does not differ with me from the time of prayer and in the noise and clatter of my kitchen, while several persons are at the same time calling for different things, I possess God in as great tranquility as if I were on my knees."

No matter where we are, what we are doing or who we are with, we can always receive God's presence. When a prayer is on our lips at any moment of the night or day, God is near. To describe that feeling is like describing love or patience or gratitude. Pat Conroy said in his book, *The Great Santini*, "There is no other word for 'thanks' but thanks and that is not enough." Likewise, there is no other way to describe the presence of God without receiving the presence of God, and that experience is indescribable.

Fourth Quarter people, for the most part, are very familiar with prayer because our prayers have been received and answered. No matter the faith we possess, that faith calls for prayer. Even if we rarely attend church, the power of prayer has been manifested. Even though our government discourages prayer in public places, there is a chaplain of the Senate that opens each session with prayer. And if prayer is ultimately pronounced illegal across the country, silent prayers will crop up as prolific as corn stalks in the fields of Iowa.

Again, prayer is the power base for MAD Fourth Quarter people who are committed to making a difference. Prayer wrenches us out of our complacency, keeps our senses focused and our brain programmed toward finishing our mission.

So, if prayer is the balancing factor that weds giving with receiving, then prayer equalizes the two so long divided.

Fake Intentions

In the fourth quarter, when a football team is losing, the quarterback often whispers to his team that it's time for a fake field goal, or a fake punt, or even a false start, depending on the circumstance. These are deliberate ploys to catch the opposing team off-guard. They do this by appearing to make a certain play, then quickly shifting their positions to execute their fake play. To fake is to fool. To fool is to deceive. To deceive is to undermine or eradicate true intentions.

Intentions are tricky things. So let's start with a definition. An intention is "to have in mind a plan, to direct the mind, to aim."

That said, all our actions then are preceded by intentions. Every move we make begins with an intention. I sit down to type, my intention is to type. I am going to take a shower. That is my intention. I intend to pick up that paper on the floor. Whether I am aware of an intention coming before my actual action, or not, the intention is always there. What is tricky about intentions is deciding which is more important, the game or winning? Is our intention to win or is our intention to play the game to win? A fine point is put on this because intentions are often misused and abused.

This means we cannot go willy-nilly through life reviewing our actions without first reviewing the stimulus which caused those actions—our intentions.

When I wrote the first sentence of this book, I stated, "I am on a mission and I want others to join me. My intention was to recruit other seniors, like myself, into being proactive in their retirement years. I was appalled at so many of my friends, who were satisfied with sitting out the game, as non-contributors to society, especially those who had so much to give. My intention was to someway inspire or motivate these friends to give back some of what they have been given. This is still my intention.

I was at the doctor's office today getting my six-month checkup. My doctor brought me into his office, sat me down and told me that he was retiring in December and that he would be transferring my case over to one of his associates. After a brief discussion of my disappointment in his leaving, I asked him what he was going to do when he retired. As active a man as he is, I knew sitting around was not going to satisfy him for long. He mentioned enjoying his retirement home in the Hill Country and his grandkids. I pointed out that even grandchildren grow up and leave the grandparent's nest. He then confessed, "I may do some missionary work." I asked what kind. He answered, "Going to Indonesia as a surgeon." That caught my attention, and I told him about my book on the fourth quarter and to please let me know what he decides as I would love to have him as one of my 'still in

THE FOURTH QUARTER

the game' examples. I am confident this beloved doctor will follow through with his missionary work. His intention, when lived out, will make a huge difference. I am proud of that kind of Fourth Quarter person.

However for some, intentions alone will not get them what they want. Like my cell phone calls, some good intentions are suddenly dropped for no good reason other than the wire is dead. People lose interest or are distracted. Having special interests or ideas cannot stand alone, without motivation to spur them on. The intention to activate an idea has to be stronger than the interest or the idea will soon be found wanting. Intention is the power, interest and ideas are the tools. Motivation and desire complete the process.

Steve Pavlina, a coach in personal development, says that "intentions without desire have very little power to manifest. If I don't really, really, really want it, there's no point in intending it."

Have you ever been in a situation in which you were scheduled to do something you really didn't want to do? Immediately you are in conflict. The intention is there, but not the desire.

Last month my husband was scheduled to have an eye operation. The eye doctor had convinced him that surgery was necessary. The date was set and the operation was scheduled but during a pre-opt test, his EKG exam showed a slight irregularity. To proceed with the operation, he had to have his cardiologist agree to the surgery. At the cardiologist's office, another EKG was taken and the doctor found the same irregularity. The cardiologist said that since the eye surgery was low risk, he could either give my husband permission, or if my husband preferred, he could ask the eye doctor to postpone the surgery until further tests were completed. My husband, who already knew that he really didn't want to have the surgery, suggested that his cardiologist call the eye doctor and postpone the scheduled surgery. My husband had every intention of fulfilling his appointment, but when he realized there was a chance to postpone it, he was all in favor.

Whether the intention is good or bad for the Fourth Quarter people is not the point, but whether the intention is a pipe dream or a true mission that can be accomplished. When I send a manuscript to a publisher for evaluation, my private desire is that the book will have such an impact that it will snap up as the next best thing since Oreos, selling millions of copies. That's a big pipe dream. When I come down to earth, reality hits me in the eyes. It's not going to happen. However, my intention, regardless of how many or how few copies are sold, or why I wrote the book in the first place, is to launch an idea worthy of followers. If I can inspire even one person to find and pursue his or her purpose, then my intention is not a daydream.

Principles of the Game:

The Empowered Mind by Gini Graham Scott

Gini Graham Scott considers receptivity our inner radar, and being in a receptive mode helps us tune into our inner knowledge and understanding. She adds, "To use this inner radar you first have to pay attention and notice it. It must be cultivated, or like an unnourished plant, it will start to wither and die, but once you start recognizing it, it is an extremely valuable tool."

Being receptive is an active exercise, not a passive one. Like a football wide receiver, a truly receptive person has to be prepared. Lacking preparedness can sometimes make us vulnerable to surprises, to criticism, and even to failure. Not all passes are completed. That is why a true receiver gives himself permission to be out there, to be involved in the hard tasks, the difficult situations and even in the impossible causes. That is the glory. Overcoming the barriers to win the game is the game itself. There would no reward without the conflict.

But as Scott points out, as difficult as being receptive might be at first, it becomes, with practice, one of the most valuable tools at our disposal. When one gives himself permission to be receptive, a hemisphere of golden opportunities arises within earshot and eye range, and we perceive opportunities in direct relationship to our 'calling.' Being receptive is a doorway to finding and acting upon a calling. Believe me! You cannot give anything or present anything or offer anything that is not yours and nothing is yours until you have allowed yourself to receive, or to put it as Jesus might have said, until you have been born again spiritually and find yourself warm and comfortable in a receiving blanket.

Other obstacles to receptivity are close mindedness and a sense of unworthiness.

Being closed-minded, as an obstacle to receptivity, is difficult to change. Like the saying goes, 'my mind is made up, don't confuse we with facts.' We all know people like that and in today's world, when the internet spits out a plethora of information, with little verification as to fact or fiction, it takes some careful attention to change a person from being adamant to being open-minded. Close-minded people have an aversion to listening to anyone who does not think as they think. This is both limiting and unfortunate. The world has too many variations and dimension, too many positives and negatives, too many new ideas and too many interpretations of any subject for someone to speak in an emphatic manner about almost anything. Death and taxes are still the only thing we can say is for sure. Right?

Not being a professional in personal or emotional disorders, the only thing I might say about an inferiority complex is that it is generally brought about by being non-receptive to the positive things in one's life—positive people, positive events, and positive insights. We douse ourselves with feelings of insecurity when we see the world as half empty or incomplete, unfair or dissatisfying. When a negative reaction is one's first reaction, receptivity is stifled and rejected.

There are people in the world who are positive and there are those who are negative thinkers, and you probably know which way you tend to think. And if the adage is true that what we are as a young person will be more so as we grow older, then it behooves us to honestly reevaluate who we are. If we are cheerful, fun loving, generous, kind, and enjoyed living in the early years, we can reasonably expect to continue to enjoy these attributes as a senior citizen. However, if we were suspicious, fearful, disbelieving, and non-trusting as a young person, the chances are we are now considered a curmudgeon. My contention is that most curmudgeons will not pick up this book.

The MAD Fourth Quarter people who are openly and cheerful receptive and maintain a sense of humor are people everyone wants to be around, like Jane who sees everyone as loveable, or Bob who embraces the world with an intellectual certitude, or Janet whose refreshing demeanor blesses us every day, or Roxie who brightens our coffee hour with a winsome wit.

From the Sideline

For over forty years, I have been aware of being receptive. I have read as much as I could find on the subject, but nothing that I have read equates to what I have learned by engaging in receptivity. Early on, reading William James' *The Will to Believe* had helped me think through the process of being receptive. I learned that I am not the current or the power, but the wire—a conduit that allows the power to flow through me freely. When an electrician checks out the connective receptacles of electric current, he speaks of a live wire or a dead wire. A live wire makes proper connections, while a dead one stops the flow of the current. I then asked myself the question, am I alive to being receptive to God's current or am I dead wire? Live wires sizzle with excitement, anticipating any future possibilities. We are alive to opportunities that seek to connect, and we become transformers or converters, recasting the current into power. According to James, "Aliveness means willingness to act irrevocably."

Willingness, then, is the operative word. "You gotta wanna," as they say. Since I am merely the wire and not the current, I must be a willing and responsive wire in order to spark the proper connections. And it follows, as night follows day, that connecting the voice of God to the impulses of the heart provides the enlightened power for all wide receivers.

I went to a concert the other night. I have been too many concerts, but that night, I approached the evening with a new resolve. I would listen differently. I would attempt to pick out individual instruments and listen for its distinct contribution to the overall performance.

When an orchestra is playing in full complement, it is almost impossible to distinguish individual players. The maestro directs his orchestra to play as one, to allow the composition to speak rather than the separate players. His ultimate goal is to bring his diverse players, with different sounding instruments, playing different notes, into one massive mountain of blended harmony.

But on that night, I wanted to see if I could detect the piccolo or the oboe, or if I could distinguish the French horn from the cello. It was not easy. When every instrument is playing at the full throttle, searching out one isolated instrument is like hunting for a four-leaf clover. It's possible, but difficult. I closed my eyes and listened. Soon, I could detect the haunting sound of the French horn, then the poignant hum of the oboe. I realized how each individual instrument contributed to the total effect of the entire orchestra. The result was amazing. No soloist stood out, but as the company of musicians played their individual scores as written, the concerto rang through the hall with harmonious beauty. Had I not been receptive, I would have failed to fine-tune my ears and missed an extraordinary experience.

Now, I'm sure that when I go to another concert, I can already discern the roles of the different instruments. When once the orchestra seemed only to play a swarm of notes, the musicians will now become individuals for me with a mission to enhance and perfect the concerto or the opus. No wonder it's said, 'music hath charm.'

An End Run

I confess I am one of those people who hate to ask a favor. Others, too, have the same aversion. Lumps form in our throats when we start to ask a favor, either because we consider it demeaning and beneath us, we don't want to ingratiate ourselves, we don't like to inconvenience a friend, or we fear being turned down. We can handle this, we say to ourselves, so we avoid asking. Not that I think asking is a sign of weakness, but more a sign of being needy. Through the years I have met people who struck me as needy, and I didn't want to be one. I also hate to be rejected. Early in thinking about the content of this book, I asked my fellow coffee goers to respond to a questionnaire I had prepared. After one of the group refused to comply, others followed one by one. This rejection temporarily sabotaged my interest in writing this book and for some time I delayed starting it. My entire formula for the book was shot down in a wink. So I am now reluctant to ask questions which might be perceived as uncomfortable.

Consequently, I learned that asking is often risky, and I had to ask myself, was the risk worth it? As a wide receiver, I waited and listened, then it came to me I could reverse my position and make an end run. I would still use some views of the coffee group but with restrictions and reduction of participation. This experience taught me not only to be careful in asking a favor, but even more careful about the content of the favor. This group was fearful of self-disclosure in print and rejected exposure in that manner. Their trust factor was weak and their risk factor even weaker, but now I understand and respect their feelings.

However, I believe I need to overcome my dislike of asking favors, if for no other reason than to level the playing field. As reluctant as I am to ask, I am open and encouraging of others to ask me. So what kind of logic is that? I am not talking about the everyday type of asking, like 'please pass the salt.' I'm talking about asking when it costs both the giver and the receiver something. When I ask my friend, Annie, to read my manuscripts for content errors and writing flaws, I am exposing myself to criticism, thus endangering my self-esteem, while at the same time I am costing my friend valuable time from her own work, and accepting her expertise as well as imperative corrections. But I have learned that when a person truly asks, it sets up the possibility for an unexpected gift.

The well-repeated Biblical verse, "Seek and you will find, ask and it shall be given, knock and the door will be opened," is for others, not ourselves. Secretly, we believe asking is a sign of weakness that might endanger our stellar reputation. A person's pride or vanity often stands in the way of humility. When pride rears its ugly head, receptivity ceases and creativity is lost.

When I ask of God, He doesn't refuse or embarrass me. He may not answer in the matter I might like, but the fear of being rejected is not there. Going to God, for me, is safe. He receives me without question. I cannot imagine God not being receptive to anyone.

A vivid and unpleasant memory makes my point. I was in college and taking a psychology course. Test time came and I took my little blue book into class expecting to ace the thing. However, I struggled with the answers and failed the test. The next day, I flounced myself into the professor's office and said indignantly, "You did not ask a single question for which I knew the answer." He responded, "I didn't want to know what you knew. I wanted to find out what you didn't know."

I will never forget that answer. He wanted to know what I didn't know! Heavens, that's an endless string. I was furious. But, when I settled down, I gave his answer considerable thought (as you can see I still remember the entire incident). When I understand the thought behind his words, I realized that what he was really telling me was that I had not been receptive to his style of teaching. His questions had not come from the textbook. They came from his lectures. I had relied on the wrong source of communication and was not open to listening. After that embarrassing encounter with the professor, in time, I became a better listener. I decided if I listened with purpose, I would learn what he wanted me to know. I abandoned the textbook and began note taking and set my mind on receptive mode. Being receptive always means listening. This is work, but it is intentional work that reaps huge benefits.

That one piece of criticism removed the wax from my ears, and I am now a listener in training. I hear music differently, I hear a lecture differently, and I hear newscasts differently. So much so, that not too long ago, I realized I had developed the art of hearing to the detriment of the art of seeing. Music means more to me than art. I cannot listen to music while I write, as so many writers do, because music totally takes over my head. I also hear what I am going to write long before the words find their way onto the page. As to seeing, although I have fairly good eyesight, art museums are not an enticement to me. One look at the Mona Lisa in the Louvre in Paris was enough, and I was out of the museum in twenty minutes. Now that I am aware of this 'seeing' deficiency I will purpose, in the future, to be more patient and attempt to learn that 'art hath charm' as well.

Giving and receiving empowers the giver. But, it is also true that receiving, as well as giving, empowers the receiver, for nothing can be given by a person who has not first received.

For a football wide receiver to become an experienced receiver, he has to practice the game. As a rookie, he first took, as it were, baby steps, and then he learned to fun fast, then to cut sharp, then to leap into the air long before he actually catches the pass.

For our MAD Fourth Quarter wide receivers, the action is similar. Once you have your goal, the goal takes over. Much like a homing pigeon, your mind is fine-tuned to that goal and the driving mechanism continues to receive the message and keeps steering us in that direction. Similar in concept to the movie, *Close Encounter of the Third Kind*, once our minds perceive a goal, everything that happens from then on has a bearing on it.

The first time I heard about the "restless leg syndrome" I had no idea what it was. A few days later I heard a television ad discussing the condition. Soon, I was utterly surprised when my doctor told me I had it. There is something about the synergy of information that compounds when one becomes aware of a specific thing. There is a process that progresses, that grows and then become full flower. In other words, the process goes from doubt—to thinking "perhaps" or "maybe"—then finally, to belief.

The mental process that moves the mind from thesis to antithesis, and finally to synthesis, is called dialectic logic. The same logic works with the process of receiving. First comes doubt, followed by understanding, and then acceptance. When one sets a goal, it is a matter of following the directions the driving force takes us and then realizing that subtle inner power will not allow us to fail. As 'love is something we do,' so is receptivity. Receptive is something we do deliberately, consciously at first, until the action becomes second nature.

I recall an incident from when I was teaching Sunday school. Christmas was two weeks away, so I used the words of the Virgin Mary as a theme for that Sunday morning class. I entitled the talk "And Mary Said." Mary is quoted only three times in scripture. The first thing she said, in response to the angel Gabriel's announcement that she had been found favorable in the eyes of God and would become pregnant was "How can these things be?" Knowledgeable about the nature of reproduction as she was, she doubted what the angel was telling her. After being told that the Holy Spirit would descend upon her and the child would be named Jesus, she realized something miraculous was taking place and she responded, "Let it be unto me according to His will." The idea was taking hold. When the full impact of her situation finally became clear, Mary issued one of the most beautiful responses in all the New Testament, she said, "My soul doth magnify the Lord...." Mary rejoiced in the discovery, and the world will forever remember her final words voiced in the Magnificat.

This is the art of receiving. At first, we doubt or suspect what is happening, and then we begin to catch on that there might be something important here, and then finally we discover what valuable tool receptivity is to our intellectual processes and our ability to accept new thoughts and ideas. Receptivity then becomes a priority.

Already in the Game

Tom Dunning is a truly remarkable man. I have known Tom for over thirty years and there is not a more dedicated man helping disadvantaged people in the city of Dallas. Tom is now retired, but maintains the honor of being Chairman Emeritus of Lockton Dunning Benefits, one of the leading employee benefit firms in the country, a business he started years ago.

When we think of 'bridges,' most of us think of grand structures built over large expanses of water or gorges like the Golden Gate Bridge. To Tom Dunning, bridges meant something entirely different. He observed that too many homeless, out of work, mentally ill, and forgotten people were sleeping under overpass bridges. He initiated the "Bridge" project and went to work finding a building where these people could have a new, clean environment to eat, bathe, and sleep. Of course, he found such a place and moved some 150 people out from under bridges into comfortable, safe housing.

But Tom wasn't finished. When he realized that the city, as well as the state, had a shortage of trained social workers, he and his wife Sally donated $100,000 to the Forty Acres Scholars Program at the University in Austin. This was a new merit-based, full-ride scholarship, created by the Texas University Exes, to recruit students to the School of Social Work. "We believe one of the greatest needs in the state of Texas for the next fifty years is for well-educated, trained social workers," said Tom.

A quietly religious man, Tom wanted to make a difference. He wanted to give back to his community what he had received from his community—a cordial, encouraging environment in which to build a meaningfully successful business. In addition, he wanted his experience in dealing with the unfortunate in our society to carry on after he could no longer participate. Tom is in his seventies.

Many women have the *Southern Cooking* cookbook on their kitchen shelf. It's a must for women who enjoy cooking. Mrs. S. R. Dull (and that is the author's name on the original copies) was one of America's first women entrepreneurs. She started cooking for funds to help meet the financial needs of her family when her husband became mentally ill. She began by preparing cakes and sandwiches for ladies at the church and soon her business began to grow. The Atlantic Gas and Light Company invited her to initiate a program of home services to promote sales for their gas stoves. Then during World War II, Henrietta Dull served as a hostess in the Soldier's Recreation House where she became fondly known as Mother Dull.

Her success at the Gas and Light Company led the editor of the *Sunday Atlantic Journal Magazine* to hire her to write and edit the Home Economic page for the magazine. When she included recipes in her articles, requests for copies poured in from everywhere. This led to the publication of the first *Southern Cooking* cookbook—a huge book of more than thirteen hundred recipes. At the time, Mrs. Dull was over sixty-five years old. The book has never been out of print since its first edition hit the bookstores in 1928.

If what Tom and Henrietta have done inspires you, consider doing any of this:

- Calling friends and encouraging them to vote.

- Working for Habitat for Humanity.

- Preparing sack lunches for the homeless.

- Serving as a coach for a school team.

THE FOURTH QUARTER

THE HAIL MARY:
Eyeing the Ticking Time Clock

Only put off until tomorrow what you are willing to die left undone.
—Pablo Picasso

Mission in Motion

If you have ever said, "Someday I'm going to…," then, today is that someday.

You have been called to action. The time has come to make the transition from your old life to your new one. Now that you have established your calling and have the mission before you, the game is on. If you feel you are coming from behind, the advancement might be tough work. The same is true if you feel you have been given a second chance. Either way, you have made the right decision. You are going to make a difference.

The Hail Mary is a forward pass made in a desperate move to win the game, generally at the end of the half or at the end of a game. The expression began back in the early 1930's and was used publicly by two former members of Notre Dame's famous Four Horseman, Elmer Layden and Jim Crowley. Then in 1975 the term 'Hail Mary' was reintroduced by the sporting press to characterize the famous Roger Staubach to Preston Pearson pass during a Dallas Cowboy's game. Staubach told reporters, "I closed my eyes and said a Hail Mary. The rest is history, as they say."

Our Hail Mary hinges more on ideology rather than desperation. For our purpose, the phrase describes the commitment as well as the confidence to do whatever it takes to make a difference. Now we are all in the game together, we have set our purposes in motion and feel an urgency to complete them, and time is running out.

Checking the current score, so far, we have made progress in shifting our attitudes about our culture, our retirement lifestyle, and our reason for still being alive. We have agreed that we must put away preconceived and hard-nosed ideas to make room for new and revolutionary approaches to longevity and its advantages and disadvantages. We have learned that a purpose or calling is an integral part of our makeup, and has now made itself known and is waiting for our attention and involvement. We have realized or have been reminded that our spiritual resources come from God and we are now including Him in our future plans.

I don't have to take a poll as to what retiree would truly like to do in retirement because bestselling author, Hyrum A. Smith, already has. Here is what he found when he asked the participants in one of his workshops what they would really like to do if time and money were no object.

I want to—Build furniture for my house that would last a generation.

I want to—Learn Chinese.

I want to—Save a million dollars.

I want to—Study history, learn to draw, have fun painting, and learn to knit.

THE FOURTH QUARTER

I want to—Eat every meal with friends and family.

I want to—Bicycle across the country, meeting people, and recording their stories.

I want to—Get enough sleep.

I want to—Run the New York Marathon.

I want to—Take flying lessons to become a pilot.

I want to—Build my dream house by hand, utilizing only myself and my wife's talents.

I want to—Volunteer my time working with children in need.

I want to—Go back to college.

I want to—Be a character actor on Broadway.

I want to—Ask all the questions I might normally be afraid to ask, and answer truthfully all the questions asked of me.

Were any of these your answers? They seem to be typical of a random group of people. There is certainly a variety of different answers from both men and women. Some are straightforward, others more emotional. I found several that indicated lifelong desires. They all sounded sincere.

Looking over this list several observations come to mind. No one wanted to be a farmer. No one wanted to continue doing what they were doing. Children or grandchildren were not specifically mentioned. And with exception of the house builders, the caveat of time and money was no object seemed to be totally ignored and didn't have any bearing on their answers.

I am sure Smith would analyze their answers as being normal, traditional, and not surprising. He would be right. The answers were exactly on target for the purpose of his workshop.

Each answer gratefully suggested activity, in response to the gist of the question, what you would really like to DO. I liked that. I am always for doing.

But I am also always for Being. And I think of the person who, when asked a similar question, responded, "I want to be the man I am supposed to be." Or another answer, "Leave this world better than I found it." They were so all-American.

However, there is an obvious omission in the answers. None of these responses mentioned God, faith, or church or any spiritual activity. No doubt, this was due to the setting and atmosphere. Smith's workshop was not held in a church but in a business setting. The instructor is not a preacher but a highly successful 'life manager.' And we all know that participants general respond to how and what they perceive the teacher or instructor wants.

In this list of 'what you always wanted to do,' I sensed a lack of destiny. And, destiny is what we ought to do. Destiny is a personal obligation to be fulfilled at all costs.

Richard J. Leider boldly writes in *The Purpose Project, An Incomplete Manifesto of Retirement* that purpose is essential to staying alive. "If there is no contact with purpose, there is spiritual sadness inside us—a deep disappointment—a retreat into self-absorption."

The author Harold G. Koenig also said, "Having a purpose and vision during retirement is one of the most important determinants of mental, social, spiritual and physical well-being in later life."

The situation is ripe for a Hail Mary. We must stay alive to stay in the game. And we must feel about our purpose as strongly as Roger Staubach did when throwing the football to Preston Pearson. We will overcome all barriers, obstacles, poor intentions, and even physical limitation to complete our mission.

So strong is the power of individual people who makes the connection with God that our life begins to soar on eagles' wings, and if we follow our purpose to the end, we will make a difference.

Principles of the Game:

Notes to Myself by Hugh Prather

Hugh Prather wrote this book at age 32 with an eye peering into the hidden wholeness of one who thinks beyond his years. This is the first of his many books and I have had this copy since 1970 because of these words:

"Often the desires that I think are for the future are based on unrealistic concepts of myself that I want to fulfill. I want to work out a theory of reality based on precognition—is this a desire to be myself or a desire to fulfill some wishful thinking of myself? I am all that I am in the present. What I wish I were or think I ought to be has to be looked for in the future."

And again: God revealed His name to Moses, and it was: I AM WHAT I AM.

We are at the point now where MAD Fourth Quarter people are renewing their positions. We have made a major decision, a choice, if you will, that will define us for the future. Some choices concern where to live, how to put our talents to the best advantage, what we want our legacy to look like, and how we view our own immortality. Some choices are physical while others are intangible, dependent on philosophical and spiritual considerations.

The power of the individual is now tantamount to success, as it always has been. So let's reawaken and realize that even though our physical powers are diminishing, our intelligent and creative powers have never been more focused. We are in the wiser stage of life acting on a wider screen.

King Solomon of the Old Testament comes to mind. He was just a lad when he found himself King and ill-equipped to rule. So he prayed. God said to him, "Ask what I shall give you." And Solomon reiterated that he, as the son of David, was now king and didn't know how to go in or come out and with so many people to rule he needed an understanding heart to judge what was good or bad. God reached into his gift bag and said, "Since you have not asked for a long life or wealth for yourself nor have you asked for death of your enemies but for discernment in administering justice, I will do what you have asked." The Hebrew Bible adds, "The whole world sought audience with Solomon to hear the wisdom God had put in his heart."

Solomon, as you know, became the author of much of the Bible's wisdom literature, including the collection of Proverbs, Ecclesiastes, and the Song of Solomon. He is a perfect example of what one person can do who makes the right choice.

History bears this out. We can enumerate many individuals who changed the world, and thus changed our lives, our culture, and how we live today. There is no better example than Jesus Christ. Of course, you say, but he had God behind him. Yes, he did, which is precisely the point. Individual persons, throughout the ages, have contributed to our well-being today, like Johannes Gutenberg and the printing press, and Martin Luther and the Reformation.

More recently and in our time, there was John Glenn the astronaut, General Dwight Eisenhower, Gandhi, and even Todd Beamer. Think of the men and women in technology who have revolutionized the way we communicate. Think of the researchers in medicine and biochemistry who have spent their lives developing medical procedures and disease cures that prolong our stay here on earth. All of these individuals, many of whose names we will never know, have made our days brighter, healthier, wiser, and easier. Their contributions will last far beyond their years.

Consider Dr. Jonas Salk and his discovery of the polio vaccine, Tom Watson with IBM, and Jean Nidetch's Weight Watchers. What contributions these are!

These are outstanding accomplishments and we have no idea as to any of these people's spiritual connections. Some may have felt they were following God's plan, others may have simply been doing their jobs, when something marvelous happened and destiny was assigned to them. What I am sure of is that God was behind their discoveries.

As grand as these discoveries may be, and as helpful as they continue to be to all of us, the smaller contributions also change lives. Those of us who know we will never go down in history as an Einstein or an Edison, should know that whatever our purpose in life is, that purpose has its place in the grand scheme of things. We are not wise enough to know God's grand plan or judge what is worthy or not; we only know that when we give ourselves purposefully as God will give us the wisdom and strength to do it. Roxie said, "After you asked me about my destiny I gave it some thought and realized that I had not consciously been aware of my purpose. Then I thought of the time I spend in the slums of a city, providing physical therapy to people who the rest of the world cared nothing about, and it dawned on me that I might be fulfilling my destiny."

Small acts of kindness, simple nods of approval, short notes of congratulations, are truly the essence of destiny making.

I remember a story I heard years ago, when the elder George Bush was president. After he initiated his Thousand Points of Light program, he followed through by meeting some of the people whom he considered one of his points of light.

In Phoenix, Arizona, a woman went every Tuesday to a nursing home to read to some of the residents, help them with their bathing, and in general offered herself to those who truly needed her. She had been doing this every Tuesday for years and the people always looked forward to her coming.

When she got the call from the President, she was stunned to be singled out. As they chatted, the president asked if she would honor him by joining him for lunch. He mentioned the date when he would be in town.

The woman thought for a minute, and then said, "Mr. President, I'd love to have lunch with you, but that is on a Tuesday and I always go to my nursing home on Tuesday, but thank you anyway."

Small steps for man, giant steps for mankind comes to mind here. This lovely lady did not orbit to the moon, she only went down the street and history was made. This is the type of action that makes a difference and, no doubt, this was that lady's destiny.

From the Sideline

For 40 years I was a minister's wife. I loved my life. I've already told you how I liked every day to be different, and I couldn't have been in a better position than being part of a church family. Imagine being an intimate part of hundreds of people's lives all at once, from baptizing the babies, marrying the young people, and then standing beside them at a gravesite. Imagine being a part of their decision-making in business, working with recovering addicts, arbitrating divorces, and helping to reset lives on firmer principles. Then imagine standing by bedsides, praying at football games, nursing homes, even at board meetings and special events.

There was nothing routine about my life. My husband and I lived day by day in a cluster of people with sad faces and happy hearts, with problems too big to bear, solutions too hard to master, and joys too wonderful to describe. The gamut of activity and the solemnity in the private lives of others became part of our lives, their families interrelated with our family, and often, our vacations were with members of our church.

THE FOURTH QUARTER

As a Methodist minister, my husband was assigned a church so we moved as often as other corporate employees. One might think this was a disadvantage, especially for children. Moving did involve adjustments and agonies, but looking back, I realize how totally positive the process was for us and our children. Moving constantly produced friendships in many places, and more often than not, those friendships were forever.

I can say, without hesitation, that my friends are my legacy. Friends also make up my spiritual estate. Many of them are gone now, but I will leave these friends and the joint memories that go with them to my children. They are a part of my children's childhood and youth as they are part of who I am today. Each one has touched my life with an indelible marker that cannot be erased. Shared life experiences, parties, weddings, funerals, picnics, Christmas pageants, Easter Sunrise Service, vacations in the Tetons, potluck suppers, Bible studies, Holy Land trips, helping our dog Touche have puppies, playing football, watching musicals, visiting the hospital, lunching at Neiman's—all these done with friends for over 40 years crystallize into an album of autumn memories. The inner sight of it is breathtaking.

The couples part of my life ended much too soon when my husband died of a massive heart attack. In a second, my world changed. When I realized that half of me had died, I had to do something to fill the space in my heart, the emptiness in my surroundings, and the loneliness in my mind. I moved. I started a business. I started writing again. I also began attended the coffee group. Soon a new world and a new citizen began to take shape. I was 61 years old.

For the next 20 years, I left my house alone, went to church alone, ate alone, and came home alone. And again, I loved it. This was my life. During those years, 'free' was not the description that fit me. Better words were spontaneous, unregimented, and unencumbered. I was happy where I lived, the friends who surrounded me, my family who supported me, my business that kept me occupied, and having coffee with the group each morning, entertained me. Also, during those years, I served on the Board of Directors of a bank, was on the Finance Board of the Downtown Rotary Club, and was Chairman of the Board of Trustee for Perkins School of Theology at Southern Methodist University and writing a book a year. In spite of the fact that I had a bout with breast cancer, had a mastectomy and the usual round of chemo before complete recovery was obtained, I never missed an important board meeting. That was my winter of discontent. The years were piling up steadily one after the other, but I was feeling good and my age didn't seem to matter.

Already in the Game

No one can exemplify the concept of Hail Mary more than Art Buchwald. No matter that he was Jewish by birth, the concept applies. Art grew up as an orphan, joined the Marine Corps when he was underage, and spent the next few years in the Pacific Theater during World War II before he was discharged as a Sergeant. He enrolled in the University of Southern California even though he had not graduated from High School; consequently, the school would not allow him to receive a degree. (Much later, he received an honorary doctorate from the school in 1993.)

Art became a columnist while living in Paris, France and when he returned to New York he became one of the most familiar columnists ever to work for *The New York Herald Tribune*. He won the Pulitzer Prize for commentary in 1982.

What makes Art remarkable for our study is the fact that he did not allow age or illness to deter him from writing. In 2000, at the age of 74, Art suffered a stroke and was hospitalized for two months. In 2006, the Associated Press reported that Art had had a leg amputated below the knee and was staying at Washington Home under Hospice care. While he was there, he was interviewed several times, and he revealed his decision to discontinue hemodialysis, which had previously been initiated to treat renal failure. He described his decision as his 'last hurrah,' stating that "If you have to go, the way you go is a big deal." At this point, Art was still writing his columns.

In 2006, Art returned to his summer home in Martha's Vineyard to complete his book titled *Too Soon to Say Goodbye*, about the five months he spent in hospice.

In November of 2006, Art appeared on the Diane Rehm's show describing himself as a "Poster boy for hospices—because I lived."

He died the following January. That day, *The New York Times* posted a video obituary in which Art appeared and declared: "Hi. I'm Art Buchwald, and I just died." If that's not a Hail Mary, I don't know what is.

Ed Williams is a long-time friend. Chuck and I occasionally meet Ed and his wife, Martha, for breakfast. He is an engineer by profession, having built several buildings on the Southern Methodist University campus. Before that, he was in the Navy.

Now in his early eighties, Ed has a passion. When he and his wife decided to sell their home and move into a retirement facility, he had only one request. The place MUST have a workshop. You see, Ed's passion is designing and building Christian crosses. Each cross has a unique story behind it, a story pertaining to the wood, or the inlayed glass or the type of design. They are extraordinarily beautiful. He sells some, but gives most of them away. Homes and offices all around Dallas have one of Ed's hand-carved crosses on their walls. Think of how long these will be cherished and the artist who created them.

Ed is giving back a portion of himself with each lasting gift. His talent is part of the gift. I have two of them.

If Art's or Ed's experiences inspire you, try:

- Helping at a day school.

- Babysitting once a week for a home-bound mother.

- Collecting Toys for Tots at Christmas.

- Making pillows for a Veteran Hospital.

THE FOURTH QUARTER

THE FINAL SCORE:
Crossing the Goal Line with Personal Satisfaction

I am old enough to see how little I have done in so much time, and how much I have to do in so little. —Sheila Kaye Smith

Goal in Sight

If you have found your purpose and are sharing that passion with others, your score board is looking great. You are making a difference every day and are one of my MAD missionaries. But don't think you are through. The game is not over. There is still time to add points to your score. We are down to yards not long gainers. Too late for Hail Marys and too short a distance for field goals. The big plays are over. We can't give up because we have not totally completed our mission.

Now is the time to chalk up the many little things that make the world go round. The big achievements are not the only things that count. Most of us can't establish an orphanage, or discover the cure for cancer, or find an alternative fuel supply. We are not another Mother Teresa, or Rachael Carson, or Steve Jobs. But we are still in the game, because we can still give ourselves away.

Principles of the Game:

Try Giving Yourself Away by David Dunn

I have had a copy of David Dunn's book for more than 40 years. Published first in 1947, the book caught my eye and I have read it several times, marked it up extensively, and have suggested it to others to try and obtain a copy. Dunn dedicated his book to "Every man and woman who is seeking greater happiness—NOW." He believes that if people purposefully give themselves to others, happiness is the immediate and ultimate consequence. I also believe this is true.

Dunn tells how he happened to write his book in the first place. He was traveling on the Twentieth Century Limited from Chicago to New York. As he lay in his berth, he wondered where the eastbound and the westbound trains passed each other in the night. The idea of "Where the Centuries Pass," as a promotional theme or motto for the railway stayed with him all night. The next day he wrote to the New York Central Lines and presented the idea of "where the centuries pass," 'with no strings attached.' He immediately received an answer. The trains pass near a little town of Athol Springs, New York, and nine miles from Buffalo. But that was not the important message. Another letter arrived soon after informing him that his idea of "Where the Centuries Pass," would be used as the subject of the New York Central calendar for the next year.

Dunn said, "The following summer I traveled extensively. In almost every railroad station and hotel lobby I entered, both at home and in Europe, hung my "Where the Centuries Pass" Calendar. It never failed to give me a glow of pleasure. It was right then I made the important discovery that everything which makes one glow with pleasure is beyond money calculations."

Dunn gave his idea away without regret or remorse. Seeing the calendars around the world was compensation enough.

THE FOURTH QUARTER

As MAD Fourth Quarter people, we are living out of the overflow. We have surplus time, surplus mental energy, surplus ideas, and most of all, gifts ungiven. We each have the gift of kindness, understanding, listening, and, perhaps most of all, the gift of appreciation to give away.

Jim Tarr, former national chief executive of the Boy Scouts of America, always ended his letters or memos with these words, 'you are appreciated.' The ripple effect of that one phrase pulsed through his organization, offering encouragement and motivation to those who worked for him. What he didn't realize at the time was the ripple effect flowed out into the larger world and is still touching lives. After Jim died, many of his coworkers and friends reminded me of this one small expression of appreciation and told me they, too, had begun to use it. Jim Tarr gave himself away a hundred times a day.

MAD Fourth Quarter people can also show appreciation a hundred times a day if we become aware of others around us. We can thank the cashier at the grocery store for their efficiency, we can thank the postman for making his route on a hot and muggy day, we can offer a glass of water to the gardener and stop a minute to appreciate what he is doing to beautify the yard. These tiny episodes of kindness and overt appreciation are part of giving yourself away on a daily basis.

Along with providing the basic human needs to those who so critically need them, you can give to others more fortunate the gift of 'attention.' A friend used to tell me that "everyone wants love, but they would settle for attention."

Attention trumps almost all other gifts in human relationships. Everyone covets someone paying attention to them.

To truly give someone your undivided attention requires more than just a momentary eye-to-eye contact. It requires listening. Not hearing, but listening. The gift of listening is golden. When our coffee group meets, it is interesting to note who hears and who really listens. The evidence of attention can be small physical signs, such as body gestures, a wink, a nod, a smile, or even a raised eyebrow often indicates the message has been received.

There is nothing quite as satisfying to a public speaker than for someone in the audience to nod or smile in agreement. There is no other gift like it. Try giving your attention away.

Our MAD Fourth Quarter people think more deeply than others about giving themselves away and looking for new ways of giving that others might overlook. Ralph Waldo Emerson wrote, "Rings and jewels are not gifts, but apologies for gifts." This is true, but 'apologies' are also gifts. To apologize to someone, especially when unexpected, is a true and welcomed gift.

One of the most helpful gifts within our coffee group is when someone turns a negative conversation into a positive one. I have noticed this happen many times during a conversation. Someone will jump in with, 'let me change the subject' and the negativity suddenly dissolves and the conversation picks up with an entirely different tone. To spend time talking about what is wrong with politics, people, or the economy is a drag on any sustained conversation and actually accomplishes little. The gift comes when someone changes the subject and proceeds to insert a more cheerful dialogue. Roxie is our change agent in this regard. She is adept at inserting just the right tidbit of humor to breaks up the lumpy downers. Roxie gives herself away by giving us quips and snippets of humor at just the right moment.

Often the best way to give yourself away is simply by impulse. That is the unexpected gift which is called for by a situation or circumstance. When we find ourselves involved in a business setting, a gracious gift is the gesture of making people comfortable. Impulsively, we will say, 'Have a seat and relax.' Or we will announce that the meeting will not be a long one or the speech will not last more than twenty minutes. On impulse, we can turn an awkward situation into a comfortable one simply by sensing the feelings of others. Our instincts work for us, especially if we follow their lead and allow them to do their job.

When we begin to give ourselves away we learn that giving can become a hobby, and then a habit. We purposefully look for ways to express appreciation. We search for circumstances whereby we can change the situation for the better. And we never have to look far. Opportunities for giving ourselves away are on every corner, in every household, in each neighborhood, in every office, and every school yard. Where there are people, there are opportunities to give yourself away.

I personally give the gift of being on time, especially if I am the guest speaker. I learned this from my experience when inviting guest speakers myself. Being in charge of a program and waiting for the speaker to arrive is agonizing. This made me realize that by being on time, or even being early, I can relieve the chairman in charge of any undue worry. Nothing is worse than having a crowd of people waiting for a speaker's late arrival. I've been there and it's heart attack time. Being on time is a free gift, both for the giver and the receiver, as well as simply courtesy.

Try giving yourself away.

Like David Dunn's calendar, your gift, with no strings attached, will show up in many places in many forms, and will represent you better than an engraved, marble stone lying atop a grass mound.

Lastly, there is no finer gift of yourself than you. Write your memoir, because memory is a terrible thing to waste. If you are reading this, you can also write. Your writing does not have to be grammatically correct. That is not important. What is important is getting down on paper what your life is all about. Believe me, you have people in your life who are seriously interested in what you have to say about your life and how you have lived it.

Writing your memoir does several things. First, your memoir is your message to the world. This is your opportunity to detail your own experiences in the light of your obtained wisdom; to point out where you went right and where you went wrong, and what you learned from both. Interview yourself as to the kind of person you truly are, how and why you think the way you do. Write how you would like to be remembered and why you think you should be remembered that way. Voice your opinions, offer your perspectives, and issue your commentaries. Most of all, be honest. You are human after all, so use your voice to express your life with foibles and mistakes, wishes and disappointments. Be authentic, for you have a great story to tell—a story that only you can tell. The time to begin is now. The mike is yours.

From the Sideline

In 2009, something happened in my life that was totally unexpected. I wrote the following story three years ago and if there is any validity to the premise of this book, that most games are won or lost in the fourth quarter, and if those of us in the fourth quarter are going to make a difference we must be up and doing it, then this story applies. Here is what I wrote then.

> I have no date on which this began. The entire beginning is a blur to me. I wish I had a better handle on this, but at the time I was preoccupied with enjoying a good life. I was living in a great condo near Northpark Mall, was running a publishing company and had friends all around. I remember thinking many times as I walked through my condo how happy I was living there. My husband had died twenty years before and after five years alone in the house, I sold our home and bought the condominium. I was content and as far as I knew considered myself settled for life. I told many people my next move would be out the front door—feet first.
>
> Chuck Walker's wife had died only four or five years before. He owned a duplex, equidistant from Northpark

mall as my condo, and sometime in the last four years, Chuck started coming to the mall and joining us for coffee, but for the life of me, I can't remember when.

Chuck's entrance into our walking/talking coffee group came through our mutual friend, Geoff Gregory. Geoff had been part of our coffee group from some time. We first met him when he sat at a nearby table and repeatedly threatened us with his cane by jokingly punching us in the ribs. One day I told him to stop harassing us and join the group. He did.

Geoff knew Chuck through the Second Air Division Association, a group of former Air Force men of World War II. It was said that Chuck had previously met Geoff for coffee from time to time, but if that was true I never remembered seeing him. But after Chuck's wife died, Geoff insisted that Chuck join us. Again, I have no memory of that day. I just know that as natural as rain, Chuck Walker became a constant and loyal attendee to the walking/talking coffee group.

Shortly before Chuck joined the coffee group, the original 18 participants divided up into two groups between what I would like to call the readers and the non-readers. The readers were constantly trading books, talking about content and making recommendations for new books. The non-readers, no doubt, got sick and tired of the literary exchanges and began sitting at another table to enjoy their morning coffee in relative peace.

Chuck stuck with Geoff and the eight or nine of us who read, but for the life of me I can't recall when this was because I was now busy running a new business and working on my first novel. Consequently, I was unmindful of him other than as someone who joined us every morning at ten o'clock for coffee.

The following Christmas, Chuck hosted a party for the group and other friends at his daughter Suzie's house. The next Christmas, his daughter brought him straight from the airport after visiting his brother in California to Janet and Ralph's Christmas party. I remember Chuck called wanting to know directions to their home and as he got closer he called again for specific details as to the house. I remember going out the front door in an attempt to flag him down if he couldn't find the house. Chuck got out of the car. I was standing on the walkway, as he came up the walk. We kissed as if brother and sister. I thought no more of it.

Chuck then attended a Christmas party at my condo the next year along with the coffee group, other condo residents, and random friends around Dallas. He was just one of about 30, and that was all.

Then a year ago, one evening when I was having my dinner alone at a cafeteria, Chuck came through the line carrying his tray. He looked up, saw me and asked if he might join me. Of course, he could. He was someone to eat with, a break from eating alone.

I can't remember the discussion, but I do remember thinking what a gentlemen he was. He was not only courteous with me; he was courteous to the waitress. After we ate, he walked me to my car and opened the door as men used to do back in the dark ages. I was impressed.

We saw each other every day except Sunday at the coffee table, talked for about an hour with the entire group and then each of us went our merry way. Then one day, he asked if I would like to have dinner with him some night. I agreed readily as I ate out most nights as he did. People alone often find it easier and more cost effective eating out than scaring up something in the kitchen. But this is when my memory gets real fuzzy.

Our dinners together were sparse at first, nothing regular or intentional until one particular night after having dinner at Natalie's. We generally met at the restaurant where we decided to eat so we always had two cars. As usual, Chuck escorted me to my car after dinner. This time, however, as he opened the door to my car he swung me around and kissed me. A kiss I'll never forget, and I knew then our relationship was going to be more than a friendship.

On Valentine's Day, Chuck invited me to have dinner at one of the most expensive restaurants in town. Both of us dressed up and we had a glorious experience. From that night on we began eating together almost every night.

One night, Chuck asked if I was interested in Winston Churchill because he had been attending lectures at his church about Churchill. I said Churchill was always of interest to me, so Chuck ordered the DVDs which consisted of 12 thirty-minute lectures. By now our routine consisted of having dinner then dropping by his house to watch one or two of the lectures. We were both intrigued by this professor from Oklahoma University by the name of Rufus Fears. After his twelve lectures about Churchill we ordered another series by this same professor and began watching the videos almost every evening. We watched sitting side by side in his small den, sometimes taking notes and discussing the lecture, all the while our relationship was steadily developing.

In May, while we were eating at an Italian restaurant, Chuck asked if I would be interested in going to England with him in July. Either his daughter or son or grandson was accustomed to going with him, supposedly to carry the bags. Each of them had been many times and was well acquainted with the routine, Chuck's friends and the reason for the trips. Chuck is a Governor of a Memorial Trust in Norwich, England and must attend at least two meetings a year, but his kids did not want to go with him this time. Thus came the invitation that I join him.

Chuck will tell you I immediately said I would go, but that is not exactly as it was. I told him I would consider it if his daughter truly did not want to go. He said, of course, his daughter was the first choice, but if she continued to refuse to go would I then consider making the trip. When Suzie said she was definitely not going we polled some of our friends as to the practicality and feasibility of two single people making a trip together. We, of course, ran the idea by the coffee group. To a person, well almost to a person, each said 'go for it.'

And I agreed to go.

It is important to note that through all of this both Chuck and I stated unequivocally and repeatedly that neither of us would ever marry again. Being single for twenty years was not exactly a good recipe for remarriage, besides I was happy with my life. I was not lonely; I liked my life of freedom and choice. Chuck, likewise, considered himself happy and pleased with his life. He had Suzie here in Dallas and his son Charlie in Maine that took care of his every need. He was and is devoted to them, calling daily, if not several times a day, for help with the computer or various other needs. He was not thinking in any way of getting married. So up to the point of leaving for England, we were two happy people blithely living a life we both enjoyed and not anticipating the radical change that was ahead for both of us.

Before we left, there were cunning comments from our children that sent us both into fits of laughter. A week before I had to call my physician daughter and ask her for some medication for a bladder infection and she said, "You and Chuck been foolin' around?" When I told Chuck her teasing comment, we began to laugh. But then when Andrew, Chuck's grandson, advised him to "take preventative measures," we realized the kids were seeing things that we did not, at the time, see ourselves. So we continued on.

After those glorious four days in Norwich we returned to London to stay for a few more days to see plays and enjoy the city. This was my first acquaintance with the RAF Club. This is a private hotel club exclusively for air force members of both England and America. To say that this place is very British is to reserve the compliment. It is totally British which makes it all the more enchanting. It sits, unidentified as a hotel, within shouting distance of Buckingham Palace. In Texas, we would say it is across the street. However, there is a lovely park that one must walk through or around in order to view the Palace. The RAF Club's address is noted on a small plaque that is almost invisible, beside the entrance, which is how the Brits like it. They are not in the business of advertising with neon signs and glitzy canopies. If fact, if you what to go to the RAF Club you must know where in the heck it is.

London formed the backdrop of our commitment to each other. There we had the time to think about all the complex issues and reasons for either marrying or not marrying. After seeing a performance of the Lion King that first night, we marched around by Leister Square the next day in order to get some discount tickets for another evening at the theater. The day was perfect, the weather as well as the Square was so inviting that Chuck and I found a nice bench and sat there for over two hours talking about what we truly wanted. Relaxed and unhurried, we sat holding hands and making our commitment. We knew we wanted to be together for the rest of our lives and talked about the best way to proceed in that direction. We had the children on both sides to consider; we had the Social Security issue to deal with and the estate planning. We talked of where we might live, either at my place or his, or should we find a new one altogether? We hammered out issues one at a time, and surprisingly they were not as large as they first seemed. The major one left up in the air was where to live, but we were so in love by this time, that we knew things would work out one way or another. In fact, we were so giddy neither of us cared. We would have lived anywhere. The objective was to be together, no matter what.

Actually, many of our friends at the mall were ahead of us in that decision. Secretly, some suspected we might marry while in London. Of course, they didn't know that we couldn't do that because of all the English laws, but realizing that they might have anticipated this, we devised a plan. So the next day we spent the entire afternoon tracing down cheap, phony wedding rings that we would wear to the coffee group the morning after we returned home.

Flying back to Dallas, we were worse than two teenagers needing a motel room. We were so full of exciting and fun plans. Chuck's daughter was there to meet us. We had so much to tell, but were stymied by the fact that our luggage was lost. We fiddled around until the airline assured us they would find our bags as soon as possible and deliver them by next morning. Suzie took the long way home, so we could tell her the high points of our visit. We did not mention the major decision of the hour.

It was dark when we arrived at my condo, and Chuck insisted on taking my bags up. Suzie had not seen my condo so she tagged along. As I was showing her around and we arrived at my bedroom and bath, Chuck blurted out, apropos to nothing I was saying, "Suzie, we are going to live together."

I was stunned. Suzie didn't hesitate. She looked at her dad and said, "What took you so long?" When I heard that, I realized we had mastered the initial hurdle. Chuck's most precious daughter, whom he depended on for so much, was in favor of our being together. I was ecstatic. One down and four children more to go. However, we were at the stage where it truly did not matter what our children wanted, we were committed to each other.

The next morning was a bit of a rush. When I got to Chuck's house where the luggage was to be delivered, I found that the bags were not on his front porch as promised, so I called the airline. This was serious. Our fake wedding rings were in my suitcase, and we had made all these big plans. The airline said they had them and would deliver them sometime that morning. I said no. They would deliver them now. We needed them immediately.

It was now after ten o'clock, the magic hour when everyone gathers for coffee and the natives were restless. I got a call from Janet on my cell phone "where are you?" "We are on our way; give us a few more minutes," I responded. The suspense was building.

Finally, the luggage arrived. We snatched the fake rings from my suitcase, wrapped mine with a piece of scotch tape so it wouldn't fall off. Then we headed for the mall.

As planned, we walked up, hand in hand, with grins on our faces as wide as summer and made our entrance. At this point the group all rose and hollered out. DID YOU GET MARRIED . . . as there were bets on? We showed them the rings and everyone thought, indeed we had done the deed.

After much hoopla, and the discovery that the rings were not a major jewelry store variety, we told them, no we were not married, but that we were going to be married on the 6th of August, which was Chuck's 91st birthday.

It was now time to run the gauntlet announcing our intentions with the rest of the family. When we told Connie, my daughter, that we were simply going to meet with Vic, my son who is a Methodist minister, and let him do the honors privately, she immediately said, "NO WAY." We are going to have the wedding at the Dallas Athletic Club complete with dinner, birthday party, wedding ceremony and the works. Suzie concurred; we were not to leave any of the family out of the ceremony.

So we were married on August 6th in the evening.

Suzie and her family got lost.

The cake made by Laurie Knox was fabulous.

The waiters were perfect.

The friends at the mall were peeved for being left out.

Chuck had pneumonia.

The wedding ceremony was tender, emotional, and memorable as Vic stood by each of us as we repeated our vows. He then asked for the blessing of the families which came together in a roaring 'WE DO.' I think I remember the champagne was bubbly and delicious. The photographer's and Miles' (my son) pictures were memorialized in a book Suzie gave us, the first like it I have ever seen, and we were honored to show it around to friends for the next six months. No one was exempt or excused from looking at our joyous faces.

On our wedding night, Chuck was so sick he asked if I wanted to go back to my condo rather than stay with him. Of course, I would not entertain that idea. I stayed close to him all night vicariously coughing and aching with him. By Monday he had a full blown case of pneumonia.

Love and Dr. Trapp brought him safely through.

That was three years ago. Chuck was ninety-one. I was eighty-one. So talk about a Hail Mary. Marriage for me at the age of 81 to a 91-year-old man was the longest shot of my life. Most people might have thought we were out of our minds. What were we thinking to start something so radical and so unconventional at this juncture in our lives? What future did we have together? And did our marriage make a difference to anyone but us? These questions have been answered to everyone's satisfaction in the ensuing years.

I share this to illustrate we are making the most of the days we have left. We are demonstrating what two people can do even at an advanced age. We hope we give courage to other Fourth Quarter people to pull away from the comfort of home and hearth and see the world while they can. We hope to encourage others to form coffee groups and sustained friendships that will help prolong their lives. We hope to laugh with others as we laugh at ourselves when we lose the keys, forget to turn off the water in the sink, and buy too-ripe bananas. Most of all, we hope others are blessed, as we have been, with the miracle of love. Chuck calls it 'bliss.'

Remember, there is no expiration date on love, imagination, creative thinking, or happiness.

But this is not about us. It is about YOU. What are you going to do now that you know you have a destiny—now that you have a pure purpose and a clear plan? If you forfeit this opportunity, then ask yourselves these questions:

1. Who loses if I fail to complete my destiny?

2. What will people miss if I fail?

3. Will my 'making a difference' be lost?

4. What will it cost my family and society and history if I fail?

5. Is my destiny strong enough to last forever?

6. Keep asking: if I don't . . . who will?

Someone once said, "When a veteran dies, a museum closes."

That statement should apply to everyone. Everyone has a story. Do not allow your story to die with you. Let it live and be remembered by those who love you most. Writing memoirs is great fun. It is easier than you think. When you recall a certain event, that event spawns a plethora of other thoughts and then those thoughts would spawn other thoughts. Before you know it, you have already written your life's story. What a gift that will be for your children and grandchildren for years to come.

To help you get started, begin where you began—with your birth and babyhood. Talk about your parents and your grandparents. Tell under what circumstances you lived your childhood. And then add the stories your parents told you. Relate the funny things they remembered you did and said. Tell some of your earliest recollections and maybe some childhood disease you might have had. Then launch into your childhood schoolmates, troubles in school, the courses you like best, and the ones you failed. Remember your school colors, mascot, and what sports you participated. Most of all, relate how you personally felt and reacted to these events.

By now, you have gotten the hang of it. When I did my memoirs, it amazed me what I did remember and how often I had to go back and insert something I had forgotten. No doubt, this will be your experience, too.

Then as a further suggestion only, after you complete your story, do your family a huge favor. Plan your own funeral arrangements and leave the details in a handy place for them to find when the time comes. Give them specific instructions as to the name of the funeral home, the minister, the hymns you want, what you want to wear, or if you want to be cremated. Do not leave the sad details to them. Then finally, leave a note where your financial records are, the name of your bank, your financial broker, and where extra money is hidden in the house. You might even want to write your own obituary. What a gift that would be! Include your best picture if you want the announcement to go into the newspaper.

You have now completed your mission. You have left for posterity your idea or your cause to live after you, and if worthy, for others to build upon. Like a friend of mine once admitted, "I don't really care about what I have done, but I care a great deal about what I have started." The truly great edifices in this world were not made in one generation, such as the cathedrals of England or the Pyramids of Egypt. Someone had to first visualize them. Then others laid the ground work while still others applied the brick and mortar.

This you have done. You have epitomized 'forever beginning.' You have made a difference that will live long after the grass that grows around you.

"Well done, good and faithful servant."

YOU HAVE MADE A DIFFERENCE!

About the Author

Dede Weldon Casad is the author of more than a dozen books, mostly about Texas and Texans. Her new series, *Henry the Hard Drive and His Friends*, are her first books for children.

A native Texan, Casad hold two degrees from Texas Women's University and a Ph.D. from the University of Texas at Dallas. She is an entrepreneur who has served on many corporate boards.

Dr. Casad makes her home in Dallas, where she has participated in a wide range of business and civic activities. She has three children and six grandsons.

Made in the USA
Middletown, DE
10 December 2016